"[*Hurry Down Sunshine*'s] fundamental strength arises from Greenberg's insistence on facing the demons that held his girl in their dark thrall. Sally's descent and tentative return form the map for this story; Greenberg's courage lies in his willingness to follow her down that terrible path, no matter where it leads."   —*Bookforum*

"The prose is so fluid that it transports us into the author's head, making his shock, fear, and love our own."
                                        —*Library Journal*

"Deeply affecting and poetically rendered."   —*Shelf Awareness*

"A story of almost mythic power...A compelling narrative about how one family coped with madness...Tough and lyrical...Greenberg brings a true writer's sensibility to every line."   —*The Times* (UK)

"[A] moving, brutally self-examining and unsettling memoir."
                                        —*Daily Mail* (UK)

"[Greenberg] writes beautifully...[He is] gratefully and minutely observant...His cast captivates."   —*The Observer* (UK)

"The psychotic break of his fifteen-year-old daughter is the grit around which Michael Greenberg forms the pearl that is *Hurry Down Sunshine*. It is a brilliant, taut, entirely original study of a suffering child and a family and marriage under siege."
                    —Janet Malcolm, author of *The Silent Woman: Sylvia Plath & Ted Hughes* and *The Journalist and the Murderer*

HURRY DOWN SUNSHINE

HURRY DOWN SUNSHINE

A FATHER'S STORY OF LOVE AND MADNESS

MICHAEL GREENBERG

OTHER PRESS • NEW YORK

Tenth Anniversary Edition 2018

Production Editor: Yvonne E. Cárdenas

Text design: Tina Henderson

This book was set in 10.75 pt Californian.

To protect their privacy, names and identifying details of medical staff, patients, and their families have been changed. In a few minor instances, the chronology of events during Sally's hospitalization have been slightly altered.

Brief portions of this book appeared, in an earlier form, in the author's column in the *Times Literary Supplement* of London on July 14, 2006 and July 13, 2007.

10 9 8 7 6 5 4 3 2 1

Library of Congress Cataloging-in-Publication Data

Names: Greenberg, Michael, 1952– author.
Title: Hurry down sunshine : a father's story of love and madness /
    by Michael Greenberg.
Description: New York : Other Press, 2018.
Identifiers: LCCN 2018046478 (print) | LCCN 2018047808 (ebook) |
    ISBN 9781590513255 (ebook) | ISBN 9781590519813 (paperback :
    alk. paper)
Subjects: | MESH: Bipolar Disorder | Parent-Child Relations |
    Adolescent Psychiatry | New York City | Personal Narratives
Classification: LCC RC516 (ebook) | LCC RC516 (print) |
    NLM WM 171.7 | DDC 616.89/5—dc23
LC record available at https://lccn.loc.gov/2018046478

HURRY DOWN SUNSHINE

PART ONE

On July 5, 1996, my daughter was struck mad. She was fifteen and her crack-up marked a turning point in both our lives. "I feel like I'm traveling and traveling with nowhere to go back to," she said in a burst of lucidity while hurtling away toward some place I could not dream of or imagine. I wanted to grab her and bring her back, but there was no turning back. Suddenly every point of connection between us had vanished. It didn't seem possible. She had learned to speak from me; she had heard her first stories from me. Indelible experiences, I thought. And yet from one day to the next we had become strangers.

My first impulse was to blame myself. Predictably, I tried to tally up the mistakes I had made, what I had failed to provide her, but they weren't enough to explain what had happened. Nothing was. Briefly, I placed my hope in the doctors, then realized that, beyond the relatively narrow clinical facts of her symptoms, they knew little more about her condition than I did. The underlying mechanisms of psychosis, I would discover, are as shrouded in mystery as they have ever been. And while this left little immediate hope for a cure, it pointed to broader secrets.

It's something of a sacrilege nowadays to speak of insanity as anything but the chemical brain disease that on one level it is. But there were moments with my daughter when I had the distressed sense of being in the presence of a rare force of nature, such as a great blizzard or flood: destructive, but in its way astounding too.

July 5th. I wake up in our apartment on Bank Street, a top-floor tenement on one of the more stately blocks in the West Village. The space next to me in the bed is empty: Pat has gone out early, down to her dance studio on Fulton Street, to balance the books, tie up loose ends. We have been married for two years and our life together is still emerging from under the weight of the separate worlds each of us brought along.

What I brought, most palpably, was my teenage daughter Sally, who, I'm a little surprised to discover, isn't home either. It's eight o'clock and the day is already sticky and hot. Sun bakes through the welted tar roof less than three feet above her loft bed. The air conditioner blew our last spare fuse around midnight; Sally must have felt she had to bail out of here just to be able to breathe.

On the living room floor lie the remains of another one of her relentless nights: a cracked Walkman held together by masking tape; a half cup of cold coffee; and the clothbound volume of Shakespeare's *Sonnets*, which she has been poring over for weeks with growing intensity. Flipping open the book at random I find a blinding crisscross of arrows, definitions, circled words. Sonnet 13 looks like a page from the Talmud, the margins crowded with so much commentary the original text is little more than a speck at the center.

Then there are the papers with Sally's own poems, composed of lines that come to her (so she informed me a few days ago) like birds flying in a window. I pick up one of these fallen birds:

> And when everything should be quiet
> your fire fights to burn a river of sleep.
> Why should the great breath of hell kiss
> what you see, my love?

Last night at around 2 A.M. she was perched on the corduroy couch writing in her notebook to the sound of Glenn Gould playing the Goldberg Variations in a continuous loop on her Walkman. I had come home late after celebrating the completion of yet another hack job in my capacity as a freelance writer: supplying the text for a two-hour video about the history of golf, a game I have never played.

"Aren't you tired?" I asked.

A vigorous shake of her head, a cease-and-desist hand gesture, while the other hand, the one with the pen in it, scuttled faster across the page. Stinging rudeness. But what I felt was a pang of nostalgia for that period in my own life when I did something similar with the poems of Hart Crane: looking up all those alien jazz-blown words, immersing myself in the sheer (and to me virtually meaningless) energy of his language. I hesitated in the living room doorway, watching her ignore me: her almond-shaped Galician eyes, her hair that doesn't grow from her head so much as shoot out of it in a wild amber burst, her hunger for language, for words.

These studious nights, I am convinced, are the release of frustrations that have been building in her since the day, almost nine years ago, when she entered first grade. It may be for the sake of symmetry that I think of that as the day Sally's childhood faded, like the frame in a silent movie where light shrinks to a pinprick at the center of the screen. But that was the way it seemed. She wasn't learning to read, but her difficulties went deeper. The alphabet was a cryptogram: *R* might as well have been a mouth of crooked teeth, *H* an upended chair. She had as much success reading *The Cat in the Hat* as she would a CAT scan. The trick of agreement, of shared meaning, upon which most human exchange is based was eluding her.

It pained me to see this submerged look come over her, as if she had lost her sense of joy. And yet the same words that her eyes could not decipher on the page, her tongue, freed from the fixed symbols of language, mastered with a deftness that allowed for puns, recitations, arguments, speeches, if she deigned to deliver them—all attesting to a bewilderingly sharp intelligence.

One day when I went to pick her up at school, the entrance was mobbed with reporters and news crews. A girl in Sally's class had been murdered by her father. With a jolt, the crime reawakened me to the fragility of my six-year-old daughter, the more so because the killer, Joel Steinberg, and I shared a rough physical resemblance. We were both Ashkenazi Jews—same coloring, same height, same glasses. Tribally, I felt implicated in this crime, guilty by affiliation. In the demonic way that once-unimaginable occurrences have of making their replication inevitable, I felt that Sally and I had been hurled into a new level of danger: in America, Tevye's great-grandchildren were murdering their daughters.

I pushed through the news crush and found her standing in the middle of the throng holding a classmate's hand. A reporter had thrust a microphone at the girls, fishing for reactions. Sally's eyes rolled up at him. Her coat was on backward, her shoelaces untied. Her barrette was dangling uselessly from her hair like an insect that got caught there. I gathered up the girls and shoved a path through the crowd.

It was around this time that Sally's mother and I split up. We had met in high school and our divorce was like the overly delayed separation of twins: necessary and wrenching. After the upheaval of those months, Sally and I drew closer. I became her advocate, tediously defending her to her teachers, to other parents, to members of our own family flummoxed by the chasm that existed between the way Sally and most everyone else saw the world. Isn't this chasm the very place where imagination thrives? I argued. Isn't it the expression of her access to that sublime region of the mind where none of us matches up ever?

"You're as bright as the rest of them," I assured her. "Your intelligence is native, it's inside you, just get through these years, life will change, you'll see."

And it did change. We traipsed to learning lab, to afford-able specialists at a community center in Chelsea. Admitted to Special Ed., she studied rudimentary word sounds and numbers with the tenacity of a scholar trying to learn a lost language. She seemed to be fighting for capacities inside herself that would die if she failed to crack this code. She suc-ceeded and, seizing on the confidence this inspired, was returned to "the mainstream," a success of the system. Here the going got rough again, but my promise that sooner or later her dormant talents would spring to life had become credible.

And now it was happening! Bach, Shakespeare, the bub-bling hieroglyph of her journals . . . If she's up all night it's because she's savoring every minute of victory after the trials of those years.

I leave the apartment and head downstairs, five flights through a series of paint-gobbed halls that haven't been mopped since anyone in the building can remember. July 5th. Independence Day weekend. The Village feels like a hotel whose most de-manding guests have departed. Those of us left behind know who we are: the sideman, the proofreader, the lady in the straw hat with plastic grapes dripping from it who saves neighborhood dogs . . . With their owners on vacation, the burnished townhouses look comatose. Bank Street has suc-cumbed to a state of slow-motion splendor.

I walk toward the coffee shop on Greenwich Avenue where Sally likes to hang out in the morning, then almost collide with her as she rounds our corner. She seems flushed, annoyed, and when I routinely ask her what her plans are she turns on me with a strangely violent look that catches me off guard.

"If you knew what was going through my mind, you wouldn't ask that question. But you don't have a clue. You don't know anything about me. Do you, Father?"

She rears back her sandaled foot and kicks a nearby garbage can with such force its metal lid clangs to the ground. A neighbor from across the street raises his eyebrows as if to say, What have we here? Sally doesn't seem to notice him or care. There's something oddly kinetic about her presence, though she's standing still, staring at me, her fists clenched at her side. Her heart-shaped face is so vivid it alarms me. It occurs to me, not for the first time, that I'm out of my depth with a daughter. I grew up one of five brothers in a demi-monde of half-wild boys. My father spent most of his life dealing scrap metal from a warehouse near the waterfront in Brooklyn. In our home the feminine side of the world was almost nonexistent.

When she goes to kick the can again, I place a hand on her shoulder to stop her. Irritably she shakes me off.

"Do I frighten you, Father?"

"Why would you frighten me?"

"You look afraid."

She bites her lip so hard the blood goes out of it. Her arms are trembling. Why is she acting this way? And why does she keep calling me Father in this pressured, phony voice, as if delivering stage lines she has learned?

Our neighbor Lou approaches with her even-tempered sheepdog. A welcome sight. Lou's fondness for Sally dates back almost ten years, when she noticed her instinctive feeling for the vulnerable beings of this world. The more helpless a person, the more Sally poured out her heart to him, sitting with stroke and Alzheimers victims outside the Village Nursing Home, delivering a slice of pizza to the drunk sprawled on Seventh Avenue. Her strongest empathies were reserved for babies. An infant to Sally was an object of reverence. It was as if she understood how easily their lives could be shattered, in some watery moment before memory perhaps, when, on a molecular level, the temperament that determines fate is formed. Given the chance, she would hold a newborn in her arms for hours. It was an affinity I sometimes worried about, as if what she really saw in those babies was the key to some fugitive force in herself that she needed to hold onto and repair.

Lou would have none of that. "You know what *naches* is? Well, you have it in that girl. She's a giver, Michael. In a world of grabbers and shitheads, she gives."

Which is why Lou's behavior now is so disturbing. She waves to us from down the street, draws within ten feet and pulls up short. Catching an eyeful of Sally, she thrusts out her hands as if to ward off some evil spirit, yanks the leash on her sheepdog, and hurries away.

Her retreat leaves me dumbstruck. Yet Sally seems unfazed. Her normally warm chestnut eyes are shell-like and dark, as if they've been brushed over with lacquer. From lack of sleep, I assume.

I ask her if she's okay.

"I'm fine."

And I think: Lou must have thought we were having an argument and didn't want to intrude.

"Are you sure? Because you seem pretty tense. You haven't been sleeping, and I've hardly seen you eat all week."

"I'm fine."

"Maybe you should take it easy tonight, lay off the Shakespeare for a while."

She presses her lips together in an explosive clench and gives a shuddering nod.

In the afternoon I meet a friend who is visiting from out of town. We catch up over a few drinks and on our way to dinner pass my building on Bank Street. A police car is double-parked outside, empty, its lightbar dark. There is such an air of tranquility on the street that it doesn't occur to me something might be wrong. A slow night, the cops must be cooping; or else they've dropped in on the guy whose Doberman pinschers are a perennial source of complaint with the neighbors.

We continue on to the restaurant where Pat is waiting for us amid a roomful of vacant tables, each with a lit candle cup at its center.

Over dinner Pat and our friend hit on common ground: each is stepparent to a beautiful, unruly daughter. They both have tales to tell: theatrical suicide threats, splattered vats of coffee, the bread knife that sliced flesh from a hand.

"My wife's daughter is the love of her life," he jokes. "I'm just the mistress."

Pat gamely agrees. "It's like living in a bad folk tale. The evil stepparent. Last in line for affection and the first to be demonized, overruled."

In fact, most everything about Pat's relationship with Sally contradicts the evil stepmother cliché. She agonizes over Sally's schoolwork, lives at the mercy of her moods, and counsels her about the potential catastrophe of charging into womanhood prematurely—warnings that Sally clearly hungers for even when she mounts a token resistance. None of this, however, has been able to resolve one of the ongoing dramas of our household: Sally's refusal to believe Pat's devotion to her is sincere. The obstacle, as Sally sees it, is that Pat will never love her as she would a biological child—not physically, not emotionally, not ever. She is alien to Pat's body, therefore alien to her heart. Our counterarguments (that the umbilical cord is not the only means of maternal attachment; that the connection between her and Pat is all the stronger for having been forged out of the real circumstances of their lives; and, finally, that she already has a biological mother) serve only to increase Sally's gloom. "Don't bullshit me, don't even try," she says bluntly. "It's a natural law."

After dinner, it's a three-minute walk to Bank Street where we say good night to our friend and start climbing the stairs.

Sally is asleep on her loft bed, more peaceful than she's looked in days. Her small painted toes hang over the edge of the bed, and her right foot—the one she smashed against the garbage can this morning—is slightly swollen.

Beside her is her friend Cass, who is spending the night, also asleep, sweating lightly.

I go into the kitchen and notice the knives are not in their usual spot on the counter; they've been moved to the highest shelf behind a set of rarely used dishes, each blade in its slit of the butcher block rack, black handles turned toward the wall.

I'm trying to make sense of this when Pat says, "There's a note to call Robin."

Robin is Sally's mother. A born-and-bred New Yorker, several years after our breakup she forswore the city to live with her new husband in a remote part of Vermont. Our arrangement about the children was decided along gender lines: Sally would go with her mother to attend junior high school in the country, while her older brother Aaron stayed in the city with me. In a small rural school system, we hoped, Sally might fare better than in New York's.

That wasn't the way it worked. In school she felt like a misfit again, and her relationship with Robin, always volatile, took a turn for the worse. The more Sally challenged her, the more passive Robin became. By default Sally "won" every battle (over money, curfew, etc.) until there was nothing left to fight for, and she was desperate to be rescued from her own terrifying precociousness. Robin was exhausted, at a loss, in a state of perpetual surrender. And yet the more pointless their battles became, the more fiercely Sally fought them, punishing her mother for granting her the very freedom she asked for, while all along demanding more freedom, more power, *more*—fighting, in effect, for her own misery. Inevitably, Sally fell in with an older crowd: rusted cars, coded lyrics about mangled metal and flesh, dead-end dirt roads.

Her navel turned black when she stabbed it with a sewing needle, ostensibly a cosmetic piercing. At thirteen, after two years in Vermont, she returned to live with Pat and me in New York.

I dial Robin's number. "The police brought Sally home tonight," she says.

And it falls into place: the patrol car parked outside was for Sally. The cops were here in the apartment, moving those knives out of reach, at the very moment my friend and I were blithely walking by.

"Did you talk to them?"

"The police? Yes, I talked to them. Yes I did. They said Sally and Cass were out on the street acting crazy, and they decided the girls would be better off at home."

Robin's message is clear: You used to criticize my mothering, but you need the New York Police Department to play Daddy.

We talk a little more and run out of things to say. After a pause, Robin gives a whispering, oddly seductive laugh.

"Michael?"

"Yes."

Silence. During which I can hear the pulsing stillness of her farmhouse through the wires. I picture the scene: scented candles, framed photograph of her guru, books about mending the soul. Another world.

"Is there something else I should know?" I ask.

"Not really. Just that . . . I release you, Michael. I've been wanting to tell you this, and I think now is the time. I release you. And I bless you with all my soul."

The next morning Sally has the dazed look of someone who has just crawled out of a car wreck. When I ask her about last night she collapses onto the couch and presses the heels of her hands against her eyes.

I turn to Cass, struggling with the laces of her combat boots, anxious to leave. She avoids looking at Sally and she won't look at me either, deflecting my questions with a series of shrugs and grunts.

With greater finesse, Pat manages to loosen her up to the point where she choppily tells us what happened. She and Sally were out walking, Sally talking a mile a minute, trying to communicate something weirdly urgent, biting Cass's head off when she interrupted her or failed to understand. "I'll show you what the fuck I mean!" she shouted at the top of her lungs, and began stopping passersby on Hudson Street, shaking them, grabbing their arms. When a man cursed Sally and pushed her away, Cass realized it wasn't a joke. She was begging Sally to cut it out when Sally flew into the middle of traffic, rushing at oncoming cars, sure that she could stop them in their tracks. "I dragged her back to the sidewalk, I don't know how she didn't get killed. And when the cops pulled up, she started on them. Same way. All this crazy shit."

Without saying good-bye to Sally (who anyway shows no sign that she is aware of her existence), Cass hobbles out of the apartment, her boots still untied, and starts down the stairs.

I follow her onto the landing, a rush of questions. The answer to which comes to me on its own, with the force of a total solution. Drugs. Acid, Ecstasy, at the very least some galactic ganja making the rounds.

I press Cass to admit it.

All she gives me, however, is an imploring look. "We didn't take any drugs. Can I please just go home?"

In the apartment Sally remains on the couch, far away, inert. I sit down next to her, take her hand, concentrate on it. I say her name out loud, not addressing her exactly, but as if to assert a tenuous strand of contact between us.

No response.

"She may have saved Sally's life," says Pat, referring to Cass.

But why did her life need saving?

Suddenly Sally pulls away from me, jumps to her feet, and starts pacing around the apartment. She is shivering, not as one who is cold might shiver, but with a bristling inner quake of her being. And she is talking, or rather pushing words from her mouth the way a shopkeeper pushes dust out the door of her shop with a broom. People are waiting for her, she says, people who depend on her, at the Sunshine Cafe, holy place of light, she can't disappoint them, she must go to them now . . .

She makes a run at the door.

I throw myself in front of her and she shoves me against the wall. Her strength is startling: five feet four, maybe a hundred pounds, enormous gusts of energy whistling through her like a storm. Wrestling me to the floor, she rips off my glasses, claws my face till it bleeds. Pat lets out a shriek and runs over to help me. Overwhelmed by the two of us, the stretched wire of her body slackens. I break our clinch, still guarding the door, and she scuttles out from under us, retreating to the opposite side of the apartment.

She sits on the floor under a window, and we glare at each other, panting, like animals across a cage.

Recovering her composure, Pat slides down beside her. Who's waiting for you, Sally? What do you want to tell them?

That's all the coaxing she requires. She erupts into language again, a pressured gush of words delivered with a false air of calmness this time, as if Pat has put a gun to her head and ordered her to sound "normal." She has had a vision. It came to her a few days ago, in the Bleecker Street playground, while she was watching two little girls play on the wooden footbridge near the slide. In a surge of insight she saw their genius, their limitless native little-girl genius, and simultaneously realized that we all are geniuses, that the very idea the word stands for has been distorted. Genius is not the fluke they want us to believe it is, no, it's as basic to who we are as our sense of love, of God. Genius is childhood. The Creator gives it to us with life, and society drums it out of us before we have the chance to follow the impulses of our naturally creative souls. Einstein, Newton, Mozart, Shakespeare—not one of them was abnormal. They simply found a way to hold on to the gift every one of us is given, like a door prize, at birth.

Sally related her vision to the little girls in the playground. Apparently they understood her perfectly. Then she walked out onto Bleecker Street and discovered her life had changed. The flowers in front of the Korean deli in their green plastic vases, the magazine covers in the news shop window, the buildings, cars—all took on a sharpness beyond anything she had imagined. The sharpness, she said, "of present time." A wavelet of energy swelled through the center of her being. She could see the hidden life in things, their detailed brilliance, the funneled genius that went into making them what they are. Sharpest of all was the misery on the faces of the people she passed. She tried to explain her vision to them but they just kept rushing by. Then it hit her: they already know about their genius, it isn't a secret, but much worse: genius has been suppressed in them, as it had been suppressed in her. And the enormous effort required to keep it from percolating to the surface and reasserting its glorious hold on our lives is the cause of all human suffering. Suffering that Sally, with this epiphany, has been chosen among all people to cure.

Pat and I are dumbstruck, less by what she is saying than how she is saying it. No sooner does one thought come galloping out of her mouth than another overtakes it, producing a pile-up of words without sequence, each sentence canceling out the previous one before it's had a chance to emerge. Our pulses racing, we strain to absorb the sheer volume of energy pouring from her tiny body. She jabs at the air, thrusts out her chin—a cut-up performance really: the overwrought despot forcing utopia down the throats of her poor subjects. But it isn't a performance; her drive to communicate is so powerful it's tormenting her. Each individual word is like a toxin she must expel from her body.

The longer she speaks, the more incoherent she becomes, and the more incoherent she becomes, the more urgent is her need to make us understand her! I feel helpless watching her. And yet I am galvanized by her sheer aliveness.

Spinoza spoke of vitality as the purest virtue, the only virtue. The drive to persist, to flourish, he said, is the absolute quality shared by all living beings. What happens, however, when vitality grows so powerful that Spinoza's virtue is inverted, and instead of flourishing, one is driven to eat oneself alive?

With renewed force I grasp on to what I am certain is the answer to this question: drugs. Some havoc-wreaking speedball has invaded Sally's bloodstream, prompting a seizure of violent—and, most important, temporary—proportions.

Troubling as this explanation is, under its shield Sally's delusion takes on a less malignant cast. My learning-disabled daughter believes she is a genius. Believes all people are geniuses, if we can just reignite the infant fires within us. Not an outrageous notion. The Balinese believe that during our first six months we are literally gods, after which our divinity dissipates, and what is left is a mere human being. And to the gnostics we're deities who made the mistake of falling in love with Nature, which is why we spend our lives yearning to recapture a state we only vaguely recall. What is Sally's vision if not the expression of that yearning? She has returned to her idealized instant of existence, before diagnostic tests and "special needs," before "processing deficits" and personality evaluation—before the word "average" came to denote a pinnacle beyond attainment. She has voided her past, renounced the corruption of influence, turned her back on divorce, betrayal, her mother, me . . . and who can blame her?

Sally's sitting on the living room floor, her arms wrapped around her ankles, her head on her knees, shaking slightly, but momentarily quiet. Taking advantage of the lull, I motion Pat to the bedroom where we can talk without being overheard. Here, I lay out my thoughts. Surely we can understand Sally's need to pump up her ego. Psychiatric literature is filled with such cases: low self-esteem bubbling up in a froth of exaggerated self-regard. Allowing for the distorting effects of the drugs she has obviously ingested, might not her enthusiasm be indicative of a healthy desire for emotional balance?

"If we can just get her to calm down, all this will pass, I'm sure of it. She'll be back to her old self again."

"We may have to ask ourselves who Sally's 'old self' really is," says Pat.

The blank incredulity of her voice stuns me. "What do you mean?"

"You're not going to like hearing this, but Cass didn't seem stoned to me. And I don't think Sally is either. Even if she did take something, it would have to have been at least ten hours ago. Shouldn't the effects be wearing off?"

I catch a glimpse of myself in the mirror through the open bathroom door: two strings of flesh hang from my cheek where Sally scratched me.

"I have to tell you, I called Arnold," says Pat, referring to the Reichian therapist who treated her after she was hit in the leg by a car and her career as a dancer abruptly ended. "He had one piece of advice: 'Take her to the nearest emergency room.'"

The significance of Arnold's advice isn't lost on me, especially in light of his weekly radio show where he voices, among other things, his skepticism toward psychotropic drugs and the biomedical-minded psychiatric establishment. I've heard Arnold call "mental illness" a social myth invented to silence a potentially subversive sector of the population.

"I thought he disapproved of emergency rooms."

"Not in the case of acute psychosis."

Acute psychosis. The phrase shocks me. By comparison "mental illness" sounds benign. I splash my face with water; a few pale drops of blood swirl down the drain. Then there's a ruckus as the front door flies open, Pat gives a yell, and the two of us are running down the stairs after Sally.

We catch up to her on Bank Street, speedwalking west with a forward headlong tilt. She is going to the Sunshine Cafe, she explains in answer to our repeated questions, people are already gathered there, soaking in the light, waiting for her to come back as she promised.

She turns down the narrow cobblestone alley near Charles Street and, trotting to keep up with her, I have the powerful sense of having veered out of time, into some luridly accurate painting by Bosch or Brueghel: Two Fools Chasing Madness through the streets of some walled medieval town.

A minute later we're in front of the Sunshine Cafe, a dingy lunch joint flanked on one side by a flophouse that has been converted to a hospice for people with AIDS, on the other by a pornographic bookstore with a sign in its window announcing a final liquidation sale. "Everything Must Go!" On the disintegrating pier across West Street a half dozen sunbathers are precariously sprawled.

As soon as we enter the cafe, the guy behind the counter rolls his eyes at the ceiling, like he's had the displeasure of dealing with us before. Then he proceeds conspicuously to ignore us. Sally zeroes in on the only customer in the place, a mild-looking man with a crew cut and leather minishorts, quietly working through a plate of chicken Caesar salad. She sits down and projects her face right up to him. What has brought you today to the Sunshine Cafe?

"To meet a friend, I hope."

She grips his naked, tattooed arm. "You've already found a friend. I am your friend."

He squirms away from her, startled, then visibly recoils.

Sally reads the opposite message: she thinks he's hanging on her every word. She gives him a stretched, strangely distant smile. Before she has the chance to launch into him, however, the man behind the counter intervenes.

"Get her outa here. I don't want to see her fucking face again."

I absorb the shock of seeing her through his cold glare: a pariah. My heart sinks. Our neighbor Lou, this summary eviction from the Sunshine Cafe . . . I remember a legend of Solomon: outwitted by a demon, he is thrown out of Jerusalem and the demon takes over as king. Solomon is forced to beg for food, insisting he is really the king of Israel. People take him for mad. They mock and shun him. He sleeps in dark corners, alone, his clothes filthy and torn.

With Pat's help I try to coax Sally toward the door. She shoots me a murderous look and orders me to be quiet. But she doesn't turn violent. She allows us to lead her out of the cafe, and we reverse our steps through the hot Village streets, Sally between us now, gesturing imperiously like a captured monarch on a forced march.

We resume our helpless positions in the apartment, shiny with sweat, heat oozing through the ceiling in an almost visible shimmer. Sally, are you hungry? Do you want to lie down? Would you like me to read to you? My voice sounds far away and strange, as if by dint of some self-soothing illusion I have set the clock back to when she was two years old. With each question I await a response, the slightest indication that whatever spell she is under has broken and she is the child I know again. Each time, however, her otherness is reaffirmed. It is as if the real Sally has been kidnapped, and here in her place is a demon, like Solomon's, who has appropriated her body. The ancient superstition of possession! How else to come to grips with this grotesque transformation?

Another hour passes. The day feels more and more unreal. I keep waiting for some kind of spontaneous remission—the hypnotist's snapped finger, as it were—but the likelihood of this happening seems increasingly remote. A hermetic silence surrounds us. It is as if we have been struck mute. But the mute have signs, a system of shared meaning. In the most profound sense Sally and I are strangers: we have no common language. Everything is gobbled up in the iron jaw of her fixation; there is no reality apart from it. She's gone away like the dead, leaving this false shell of herself to talk at me in an invented dialect only it can understand.

"People get up-set when they feel set up. Do you feel set up, Father?"

Her voice pierces me like a dart. She is flushed, beautiful, unfathomably soulless.

"I'm proud of you, Father. There's so much to cry about. So very much."

Only when I feel the wet sting in the scratched grooves on my cheek do I comprehend what she is referring to: she thinks I am shedding tears of joy at her epiphanies; that I have embraced her vision; that thanks to her I too have been saved.

———

By late afternoon there is nothing left to do but follow Arnold's advice and take Sally to the hospital. Far from resisting this plan, as I expect her to, she greets it with a swell of optimism as if we're about to embark on a long-postponed adventure. She'll be able to "share" her discoveries with people who are versed in such matters, experts who will understand. So we're down the stairs again and scurrying along Bank Street, the neighborhood's eyes on Sally as she broadcasts her crack-up, engaging all comers, discordant and wired.

At the Bleecker Street playground she stops, grips the bars of the wrought iron fence, and with peculiar severity contemplates the children within. She seems mesmerized as she watches them run through the sprinkler, dig in the sandbox, circle one another in their plastic cars. Her breath is shallow, quick, her eyes glossy and, for the moment, immensely sad. Sad beyond her capacity to recognize sadness ("Glory in miseria," Robert Lowell called it, writing of his own abysmal elation), what I would come to know as the mixed state experienced by those in the throes of dystopic mania.

Adjacent to the playground is a small square with seventeen silver linden trees rising fifty feet and higher from what must be the deepest tree pits in the Village. The leaves of these lindens weave a roof so thick over the square the sun can't get through, even in July. It's as dark as a cave in there, and perpetually cool, a haven for can gatherers and anyone else in need of a place to curl up and be left alone. A half dozen bodies lie fetally on the benches, while others rummage through plastic sacks, change their clothes, fry sausages on portable burners, drink liquor concoctions with names like Tequiza and Pink Lady, all with an air of bedroom leisure, radios playing low, ripe odors rolling out from under the trees.

As I ungrip Sally's hand from the playground fence, a woman from the square wanders over. I've seen her before, on my way to the bank, the subway, her sea lion body sheathed in dirt, a protective armor against sadists and thieves. I go to put a coin in her outstretched hand, then see she isn't begging for money: sitting in her palm is a dead sparrow, its tiny brown claws pointing straight up at the sky. I flinch involuntarily, while with a contradictory lurch my heart goes out to her. I look in her eyes: two shiny shellacked stones, at the center of a world that to her is the only world. How unknowable we are! I start to say something to her but the chasm between us seems impassably huge.

Eugen Bleuler (who in 1911 coined the word "schizophrenia") once said that in the end his patients were stranger to him than the birds in his garden. But if they're strangers to us, what are we to them?

Indignant, Sally hisses the woman away. "Don't let her bother you, Father, she's totally out of her mind."

After sweating it out for a while in the hospital ER, with the kidney stone, the detoxer, the rollerblader with a chipped bone, we're summoned into one of a series of partitioned modules.

"Let me do the talking," orders Sally, confident that the admitting nurse will grasp the importance of her message in a way Pat and I cannot. She starts out in the lecturing tone of a schoolmarm, primly smoothing the creases in her dress: the parody of a woman in control. Within seconds, however, speech shatters like a dropped glass.

"Are you this girl's father?" asks the nurse.

"Yes—yes I am."

"Go through those doors and make a left. Take seats in one of the examination rooms. An empty one, of course."

Following her directions, we enter a brightly painted wing, strips of yellow crepe paper strung across the ceiling, Berenstain Bears cavorting on the walls. Pediatric ER.

We find an examination room and sit tight, Sally curled up on the padded table, her head in Pat's lap, as if trying to endure the fibrillation of her brain without imploding. Afraid. Frayed. Why are you so a-frayed? she keeps asking. I repeatedly tell her I'm not afraid. Then the logic of her insistence dawns on me: she wants me to be afraid for her. I am custodian for the terror that the hollow exuberance of her mania won't allow her to feel. This exuberance, I begin to understand, is the opposite of the truth. She is beleaguered by certitude because she is certain of nothing. She thinks she's eloquent, when she can't put together a coherent sentence. She demands control because, in some interstice of her psyche, she knows she is hurtling out of control.

This realization brings me closer to her. I can't witness her disintegrations without somehow taking part in them, and, closing my eyes, I feel myself racing too, as if her flutter has lodged inside me. "I feel like I'm traveling and traveling with nowhere to go back to," she says in an almost casual whisper. Pat whispers something in return, gently stroking her hair. The gesture seems to soothe the agitated solitariness that, it's increasingly clear, is her chief terror. Sally's need to feel understood is like one's need for air. (Isn't this everyone's struggle? To recruit others to our version of reality? To persuade? To be seen for what we think we are?) I envy Pat's ability to make her temporarily believe she has penetrated her mind, but I couldn't do it myself. I don't want to enter her world, I want to yank her back into mine.

A very young doctor peeks in, talks with us for about fifteen seconds, and rushes off. "I've paged the psychiatric resident. She's on her way over."

Another forty minutes drag by. Pasty light pours down from long tubes in the ceiling. The protective paper on the examination table is shredded from Sally's tossing.

The psychiatric resident arrives: short, early thirties, her eyeglasses held together with tape. She politely asks us to leave so she can interview Sally in private.

After five minutes she emerges and leads me to a tiny windowless room, a supply closet really, crammed with IV bags, exam gloves, sterile pads, soap refills . . . We sit facing each other on folding chairs, our knees almost touching.

When did I first notice Sally was acting strangely? I tell her about her recent insomniac nights, her poem about "the great breath of hell," and the kicked garbage can yesterday morning. "She wasn't incoherent yet, you understand." And then, uncomfortably aware of how unobservant I must sound: "I have a high threshold for unusual behavior, I suppose." I immediately regret that statement too. My every utterance, I fear, will incriminate me further. But for what crime exactly?

"It's not unusual," says the resident, "for this kind of illness to break very suddenly into the open like a fever. When it happens, it's shocking, I can imagine how you must feel." I give her a grateful look, but our physical proximity makes eye contact awkward. "Sally's condition has probably been building for a while, gathering strength until it just overwhelmed her."

When I ask what this "condition" is, she gives a pallid smile. "What we call Sally's disease is not what's important right now. Certainly many of the criteria for bipolar 1 are here. But fifteen is relatively early for fulminating mania to present itself. What I do know is your daughter is very ill. I strongly recommend she be admitted so she can get the treatment she needs."

"To the psych ward?"

She nods curtly and I immediately feel myself balking. Despite mounting evidence to the contrary, I've had my heart set on a last-minute reprieve. My first line of defense, drugs, has crumbled, but why not a rare metabolic disorder, like King George's porphyria, that could be routed by a strict dietary regime? Or a glandular imbalance, the chaos of conversion that marks a girl's fifteenth year? To hear the actual verdict is crushing. But how final is it? How can she accurately make such a judgment about Sally in the space of five minutes, as if she were diagnosing a case of strep throat or bronchitis?

The resident excuses herself and returns a few seconds later with a sheaf of photocopied papers, which she hands to me.

"Since your daughter is under eighteen we'll need your consent to admit her."

She unclips a pen from her side pocket—"Risperdal" it says, the latest antipsychotic medication—and hands that to me too.

Each page is marked with an X where I am to sign my name. But if I do what will it mean? I can't conceive of Sally as a mental patient; my mind refuses to accept it. I have an idea of the treatment she'll undergo—a powerful neuroleptic cocktail, chemotherapy of the brain. I've seen the result of this cocktail, we all have. I can't imagine Sally being blunted like that: staring at the world from behind a scratched shield of plastic, the bulletproof kind you see in liquor stores and cabs.

"Give me a minute, Doctor."

"Take all the time you need."

I return to the examination room to talk it over with Pat, still hoping to figure out a way to take Sally home. A nurse is drawing her blood. When she removes the needle a single drop falls on Sally's dress: an oblong crimson stain. "Look what you've done! Clean this up! Clean it off me! Now!" She pushes the hem of her dress under the nurse's nose, evidence of her heinous crime. Her expression is homicidal, as if this blood were a smear of shit corrupting everything she's been crusading for, her purity, her vision, instantly defiled. She is trembling wildly. What Sally has been experiencing, I realize, is a fragile and horrendous triumph over doubt, and this stain somehow has brought this "triumph" into question. It's the crash to come, the worm in her rose, threatening her florid bloom. And Sally won't have it.

"Get it off me!" she cries as if her life depends on it.

"Clean it yourself, sweetheart," says the nurse. Unfazed,

she drops a tube of Sally's blood in her pocket and walks out the door.

Pat removes a paper towel from the metal dispenser on the wall, wets it, and rubs at the stain, thickening it into a pale watery blob.

Sally continues screaming.

I snap at her to shut up.

Pat raises her head, questioning, frazzled. What do we do now?

Sally looks at me for a split second as if she doesn't know who I am. Then, without warning, her voice goes soft and operatically tragic. With broad, exaggerated strokes she caresses my cheek with the back of her hand. "Poor, poor Father. Trying to get back your lost genius. When all you had to do was come to me. It was right here, under your nose." And she bursts into tears.

Accepting the truth, I complete the consent forms and thank the resident for bearing with me. No problem, she says. Just give the administrator your insurance card.

My insurance card. In the upheavals of the day I had avoided thinking about this detail: Pat recently left her teaching job and our insurance has lapsed. With no apparent catastrophe on the horizon (didn't we know catastrophe is always on the horizon?), we have been shopping for a provider for months. On a shelf in our apartment a pile of benefit booklets is gathering dust.

"No coverage? Nothing?" asks the administrator.

I turn to the resident. "Whatever the bill comes to, I'll pay it. I give you my word."

"Apparently your word is all you can give me."

She half turns from me, shivers slightly, and confers with another resident: male, also young. I feel like a fish wrapped in yesterday's want ads as he looks me over. I repeat my vow— I'll pay every penny—with stentorian sincerity this time. I hold their eyes: I'm a stand-up guy, a good father who happened to get caught in a temporary insurance gap . . .

She snaps the Risperdal pen, signs the forms, and, with an audible intake of breath, walks briskly away.

The ambulance is waiting, an unnecessary extravagance. Pat and I could easily take Sally in a cab to the psychiatric clinic ten blocks away. Now that she is officially a patient, however, standard procedure kicks in. (Add five hundred bucks to my tab.)

While the paramedics strap her to the gurney, Sally races on about her epiphanies, the piercing nature of light, the lightness of light, the genius in us all . . .

The medics lift the gurney into the ambulance and lock it down. Mummy-strapped, staring at the roof of the van, she is festive and reassured. Pat and I climb in after her. It's 2:14 A.M. The street is so still I can hear the East River, about a hundred feet away, rushing against the concrete embankment. The doors swing shut.

We glide cozily over the deserted East Side streets, no siren, no traffic laws, a thick moonless night. The ambulance pulls up at an undistinguished white brick building, squeezed between two similar 1960s eyesores. The building jogs my memory: I have the odd sense that I've been here before, but I can't place when or why.

On the fifth floor we're passed through two solid steel doors, each with a tiny rectangular eye slit. A double-locked ward.

A skeletal night crew is on duty, all female, a tight cabal. Ignoring Pat and me, they instantly take possession of Sally. They have the drill down to the minutest detail. Physical contact: minimal. Tone: brusque, commanding, but not unkind. Any authority I may have had is annulled; she belongs to them now. If the resident's tendency was to exonerate us for Sally's illness on biomedical grounds, the nurses seem to view us as vectors of instability: parental failures at best, at worst suspects for mental illness ourselves. My anxious, competing claim over Sally clearly annoys them. As far as they're concerned, the sooner we get out of their ward, the better they'll be able to do their job.

They usher Sally into a tiny shoebox of a room. A gated window, disproportionately large, looms over a narrow bed: a surrealist painting in which the dream is enormous, the dreamer inconsequentially small. I start to follow them into the room, when one of the nurses bars me with an unequivocal gesture and shuts the door. I am reminded of my stint, some years ago, as a Spanish–English interpreter at Manhattan Criminal Court. When the officers took custody of a remanded defendant, they did so with a peculiar solicitude very much like that of these nurses: careful not to damage what they have no particular feeling for.

Pat and I wait uselessly in the hallway. The place is quiet, dozens of patients sleeping their medicated sleep behind rows of beige doors. On the wall near the nurse's station hangs an erasable white board with patients' privileges posted on it. D can go out to smoke (Level 3). R can eat at a restaurant with a visiting relative (Level 5). M is under twenty-four-hour surveillance. The video tomorrow will be *A Fish Called Wanda*.

Sally emerges from her room in a thin hospital gown, snap buttons, no laces or ties. She suddenly looks ageless. The only other time I've seen her in a hospital was the night she was born. By that point in our marriage her mother and I were like two people drinking alone in a bar. Not hostile, just miles apart. Yet when Sally appeared a huge optimism came over us, a physical optimism, primitive and momentarily blind. She was her own truth, complete to herself, so beautifully formed that the jaded maternity nurses marveled at what perfection had just slid into the world.

Though she has never set foot in a psychiatric hospital, there is the tacit sense from Sally that these women understand her, she is where she belongs. She acts as if a great burden has been lifted from her. At the same time she is more elevated than ever: feral, glitter-eyed. In 1855 a friend of Robert Schumann observed him at the piano in an asylum near Bonn: "like a machine whose springs are broken, but which still tries to work, jerking convulsively." Sally appears to be heading toward this maimed point of perpetual motion. Her sole concern is to get her pen back, which has been confiscated with most of her other belongings—belt, matches, shoelaces, keys, anything with glass, and her comb with half its teeth snapped off by her potent hair. She initiates an agitated negotiation with the nurses which immediately threatens to boil over into a serious scene. The nurses confer like referees after a disputed call. Then they grant her a felt-tip marker and march her back to her room.

With assurances that we'll be permitted to visit her tomorrow, they give us the bum's rush through the double-locked doors.

In the lobby, I again experience the sensation of having been in this building before, but the memory squirts away before I can grasp it.

Back at Bank Street the air conditioner won't work: I forgot to buy fuses. Pat undresses, lies down on our bed. I lie down beside her, close my eyes, then immediately sit up, my blood pounding.

Wide awake, I go into the living room. The apartment feels like the shadow of a home, provisional, funky, bearing the merest imprint of our lives. The windows are rotted; last winter one of the panes fell out like a bad tooth, narrowly missing a man who was dropping his clothes off at the laundromat five flights below. After discovering the wood was too decrepit to accept glazing putty, I reinforced each pane with duct tape. The place is literally bandaged.

Our tenancy is just as precarious. In exchange for my below-market rent, I fulfill various duties for the building's owner, such as keeping an eye out for boiler breakdowns and appearing at city agencies in response to code violations or overdue tax bills. I am forbidden to substantially improve the apartment or even to introduce a few new sticks of furniture—the owner's theory being that to do so might cause us to start thinking of it as our permanent home. He's a friend from high school, the owner, and our Byzantine housing arrangement is the kind that New York is famous for—antiregulatory in spirit rather than outright illegal. The price of my freelancer's ticket. But at what price to Sally? I have done a poor job of concealing my anxieties, living at the whim of a man who can, by our own agreement, evict us tomorrow.

Surely she has internalized this instability at the very center of our lives.

I keep picturing her in the hospital, in that gown, gripping the felt-tip pen she fought for. The resident was right, we didn't have a choice. Yet I can't stop thinking of her as a prisoner on that locked ward, where I put her.

James Joyce's daughter Lucia once told him that the reason she was mentally ill was that he had given her no morale. "How can I give you something I don't have myself?" was Joyce's mournful reply. Lucia had been variously diagnosed with schizophrenia and rapid cycling mania, but Joyce insisted that her mental distortions were nothing more than the growing pains of a gifted girl. With a gullibility that may be interpreted as an attempt to protect them both from the truth, he accepted whatever she told him at face value, once going so far as to ban every male visitor from his home because Lucia accused them—all of them—of trying to seduce her.

One day at the Gare du Nord in Paris it became impossible to continue ignoring that something was seriously wrong. With their bags already loaded onto the train, Lucia launched into an unprovoked tantrum, screaming at the top of her lungs for forty-five minutes while her parents looked helplessly on. Shortly after, at a party in her honor, she collapsed on a sofa, where she remained for days, open-eyed and catatonic. She threw furniture at her mother, Nora, the main recipient of her wrath. She sent telegrams to dead people, lit her room on fire, and would disappear into the streets for days.

Joyce was merciless in blaming himself for her troubles. Lucia, he believed, was the victim of his monomaniacal existence. He had dragged her around Europe, living in a succession of tiny apartments and hotels, turning her into a woman without language or settled home—a rootless, polyglot soul. A feature of her psychosis was a penchant for speaking in neologisms and puns that added up to an incomprehensible, almost infantile babble. No one could understand what she said. Except Joyce. He listened to her attentively, responding with the utmost seriousness and respect, seeming to enter the garbled workings of her mind with an intuitive sympathy that often left others bewildered and embarrassed.

An irresistible notion took hold of him: that his work on *Finnegans Wake* had infiltrated his daughter's brain and deranged her. He had conceived *Finnegans Wake* as a novel of the unconscious night (as opposed to the day of *Ulysses*), a novel of nocturnal wordplay and associations that might come as close as literature can to the sealed world of psychosis, without itself being insane. Surely this had precipitated Lucia's cryptic utterances. "Whatever spark of gift I possess," he said bitterly, "has been transmitted to her and has kindled a fire in her brain."

His superstition was rooted in the almost telepathic empathy between them. He instinctively understood the scorched loneliness of Lucia's condition. Madness wrenches us from the common language of life, the language that Joyce too had departed from, or surpassed. We all fear at some point that "our" world and "the" world are hopelessly estranged. Psychosis is the fulfillment of that fear. One is reminded of the manic patient in a lie detector test who was asked if he was Napoleon. "No," he replied. The lie detector recorded that he was lying. Joyce's immersion in the workings of Lucia's mind was an attempt to rescue her from that double lie, an attempt to show her that he too spoke her language. If he spoke it then how could she be insane, or alone?

Guiltily, Joyce reversed the equation of their relationship, turning Lucia into the superior one. "Her intuitions are amazing," he remarked, though he alone was capable of deciphering them. She was "a vessel of election," an innovator, foreshadowing a new literature.

It was his last line of defense against hopelessness. In 1936, when Lucia was twenty-nine, she was carried away in a straitjacket. Joyce visited her at the hospital every Sunday, trying to cheer her up with presents and Latin phrases. But his heart was broken. His drinking increased beyond his habitual wine in the evening; now it was Pernod in the afternoon. On several occasions his wife Nora walked out on him. He begged her to stay, weeping. "I feel like an animal who has received four thunderous mallet strokes on the top of the skull," he said. "There are moments and hours when I have nothing in my heart but rage and despair, a blind man's rage and despair."

He couldn't sleep, and when he did he had nightmares, bolting awake as if he were "wound up and then suddenly shooting out of the water like a fish." For a brief time he thought that he too was hearing voices. "I can see nothing but a dark wall in front of me," he wrote, "a dark wall or a precipice if you prefer, physically, morally, materially."

He had spent three-quarters of his royalties from *Ulysses* searching for Lucia's cure, coddling her with the most extravagant gestures, responding to one of her episodes with a 4,000-franc fur coat, because fur, Joyce believed, possessed mysterious healing powers. On another occasion he secretly paid for the publication of a book to which she had supplied illustrations, so she might not feel that her life had been wasted.

"Altogether, believe me," he wrote her, "there are still some beautiful things in this poor old world." Then, scolding her for her inertia: "Why do you always sit at the window? No doubt it makes a pretty picture but a girl walking in the fields also makes a pretty picture."

Informed of his death, in 1941, Lucia said: "What is he doing under the ground that idiot? When will he decide to come out? He's watching us all the time."

At first light a car alarm starts squalling on Bank Street. On the neighboring roof an elderly man in a woman's swimsuit is lying belly up on a towel.

A little after 6 A.M. the phone rings.

"You motherfucker! Arrogant prick! I hate you. You and your fucking family. I hope you die!"

It is my brother Steve. He slams down the phone. I was supposed to meet him yesterday evening at the supermarket, our weekly rendezvous to buy his ration of food.

I dial his number. He lets it ring nine, maybe ten times before answering.

"Don't ever call me like that again," I tell him.

"I'm sorry, Mikey."

"I got held up. It was beyond my control. Answer me, Steve, how many times have I stood you up?"

"Just this once. This is the first time."

"The first time. In two years."

"You're the best, Mikey."

"The supermarket opens at eight-thirty. I'll see you there."

"You're the greatest, Mikey. The greatest brother in the world."

I'm still waiting for Steve outside the supermarket at ten to nine, gnawed by the fear that he and Sally are alike, that their conditions are connected in some hereditary way that will eventually make itself clear. But what is Steve's "condition"? He never had a full-blown crack-up like Sally's; and he's never been given a definitive diagnosis either. They called him "schizoid" in the sixties, "borderline" in the eighties . . . "Chronically maladjusted" is the term now for his hopeless middle age. I don't know anymore. I never knew. Five years older than me, he's been disqualified from social acceptance since I can remember. Maybe it was how he arrived in the world: a *shoteh*, as the Talmud would call him, a mental in-valid, the responsibility of his tribe.

He finally shows up at five past nine. He isn't usually this late, but I'm too numb to scold him. All I can think of is Sally. Can this be a version of my daughter in thirty years? Arguing against the possibility, I keep returning to the glaring differ-ences between them; but what if those differences are just varied presentations of the same disease? He looks in worse shape than last week. There are cigarette lighter burns on the tips of his fingers, his T-shirt is dirty and torn. On his cheeks are a series of tiny brownish bumps. When I ask him what they are, he says, "Insects, bugs. They burrow under my skin, mooching off me, Mikey, mooching!" As his caretaker I should be attentive to these problems. But I've witnessed his phobias for so long I don't know how to gauge their seriousness. Nor do I want to right now.

He plunges into the supermarket and commandeers a shopping cart, steering it to the aisle where the tea is dis-played. Steve's weekly ration consists of one hundred bags of Lipton's (always Lipton's), which he steeps in a thirty-two-ounce pickle jar, five bags at a time.

He scans the shelves and hesitates for a moment; then it hits him that Lipton's is out of stock. His lower lip slumps out, a crinkled pouch of disappointment.

"They knew I was coming. They knew it and they took it off the shelves."

"Who did?"

"The people who work here for fuck's sake! They saw you waiting outside for me and that tipped them off. So they took it off the fucking shelves."

"Steve, look at that guy." I indicate the man in the next aisle, crouching over a shipment of pet food, stocking the shelves. "He's not thinking about you. He's got his own problems."

I can feel him churning, fortified to reject any attempt by me to contradict his suspicions.

"We're in luck," I say, "they have Tetley's. Tetley's is good too." Tetley's, I assure him, employs the same growers as Lipton's, in the mountains of India and Sri Lanka, entire villages devoted to supplying these giant buyers with tea. "The two brands are completely alike. Believe me, you're not being shortchanged."

"How do you know?"

"I just do," I lie. "I read it in the *New York Times*."

"Okay, forget it. Just fucking forget it!" He seizes a box of Tetley's and throws it into his cart.

I follow him through the supermarket while he chooses the rest of his staples: eggs, bread, fruit, soup, a tin of Captain Black tobacco. In Aisle 4 he wraps his fist around a container of Advil. "You gotta get this for me, Mikey, I'm in such pain. It's my tongue. It feels like a blanket in a washing machine, swishing around, all heavy and wet. It's driving me crazy."

I've heard this complaint before. The swishing tongue, *tardive dyskinesia*, a side effect of thirty years of chlorpromazine and its various pharmaceutical descendants. Nevertheless, I refuse; Advil won't help. And the last time he had some he took twice the maximum daily dosage.

We pay for the groceries and go back outside, air conditioners dribbling stale water from their window berths, the river simmering two blocks away, the Village like some choked backwater town. Seething about the Advil I wouldn't buy him, Steve rests his shopping bags on the pavement. He removes his baseball cap, its inner seam dark with sweat. His skin is papery and yellow. There's a black hole where an upper front tooth used to be. His jeans are stiff with grime. Looking at him, I remember the boy who would sit for hours in his darkened bedroom two steps down the hall from mine. He was more delicate than the rest of us brothers, with his fair coloring and large timorous eyes. I remember being infatuated with his almost reptilian stillness. But what was behind such stillness in a young, otherwise healthy boy?

"We've got to wash your clothes," I say. And though I know he'll spend it on Advil, or malt liquor, or some broken toaster oven for sale on the street, I give him twenty bucks for the Laundromat.

Steve looks glumly at the money, twisting the plastic handles of his grocery bags around his fingers.

"Remember Dad used to say I couldn't hack it with people because I never tried? Well, I'm trying now, little brother, I'm trying to hack it. You'll see."

He shoots me a parting smile, picks up the bags, and rushes away up Hudson Street, his eyes darting around as if he's being pursued.

I watch him go, wondering what he means by those words, yet not wanting to find out. I'll shop for him again next week. It's almost eleven now. Visiting hours at the psych ward are in an hour.

I return to our apartment. Pat sits at the table, sipping coffee. She looks exhausted, concerned.

"I tried to get Sally on the phone," she says. "They wouldn't let me talk to her."

"Was she asleep?"

"They wouldn't say."

She has packed a bag for Sally: pajamas, a toothbrush, shampoo, slippers . . . the first innocent necessities of her confinement.

We hail a cab and arrive at the clinic, patients and hospital workers smoking in self-segregated clusters outside the front door. 11:50. Ten minutes till visiting hours begin. We wait in the lobby: gray linoleum floor, Van Gogh sunflowers on the walls. At twelve o'clock sharp a large family of Hasidic Jews comes through, a bearded man leading the way, the knotted strings of his prayer shawl hanging out of his shirt. He nods to the guard and they pile into the elevator, laden with bags of food.

Pat and I start to follow them, but the guard stops us. "We're here to see our daughter," I tell him. "Sally Greenberg. She was admitted last night."

He ducks into a small alcove and makes a call on the house phone. Then he turns to us. "You can't go up right now. Someone will be down to explain. Wait here."

We wait, standing, until the elevator disgorges a sturdily built woman, keys hanging from a leather cord around her neck, and a pin in the lapel of her jacket: "Local 1199," hospital workers union, one of the toughest in the city.

"Sally can't have visitors today," she informs us. "She's too agitated. She needs time to calm down."

"But we were promised we'd be able to see her." I feel myself enter a delayed, almost frozen zone. We've entrusted her to the wrong people, we don't know what they're doing to her, they don't want us to know . . . "We were promised . . . last night . . . when we signed her into the ward. If there had been any doubt we never would have—"

"I didn't promise nothing. I wasn't on duty last night. Like I said, she needs more time."

"How much time?"

"That's up to the doctor."

She stands with her legs planted firmly, arms crossed over her keys, the guard right behind her, in family management mode, ready for a scene.

"Then let us speak with the doctor."

"I'll see what I can do. It's a holiday weekend, a lot of the staff are off."

She presses the elevator call button and the doors rattle open at once. An empty box. We follow her ascent on the panel. Fifth floor, Sally's ward, a hidden world from which we are suddenly barred.

I sit down, stunned, the guard watching me out of the corner of his eye, as more visitors wander in: a young Asian couple, upright and handsome; a late-middle-aged hipster; a forlorn woman in a gold linen suit . . . They're all allowed upstairs. We're the only ones shut out. I try to picture Sally's ward: the double-locked steel doors, her shoebox of a room, the erasable board with each patient's status: Sally Greenberg. No Privileges. No Visitors. Level Zero. At the nadir of madness.

Finally the doctor comes down, late forties, with the vague air of futility that I would come to recognize in many psychiatrists who have been at it for a while. He explains that he's only filling in for the weekend, long-term decisions about Sally's diagnosis and treatment will be made when regular staff returns to work on Tuesday. Then he answers our primary question, our only question really.

"She's in isolation. What we call the Quiet Room."

"You mean you've locked her up," says Pat.

"She's not unsupervised. Staff looks in on her every fifteen minutes. It's for her own good." Appearing to wince at the cliché, he sits down next to us on the edge of a chair, less officious than sad, an old hand at delivering bad news. "As soon as she works through her current phase she'll be permitted to join the other patients. That may require a few days, or only a couple of hours. I wish I could be more exact."

Permitted. Required. The language of punishment. Of custodianship. My heart sinks. How much worse than last night can she be? Where is the end point? My daughter in isolation, that ancient place of confinement, descendant of dungeons and barred holes in the ground. My only recourse is to revoke my consent to hold her. But can we really take Sally home? I imagine Pat and me marching her through the lobby, into a cab. Then what? We have no isolation room, no training, no sedatives or meds . . . The blunt weight of the fact stops me cold: we need this place.

I ask for the chance to see her. "Not a visit," I explain, "just to look at her, to assure ourselves she's okay."

"I'm sorry, policy won't allow it." He shrugs ambiguously, lowers his eyes. "You may find this hard to believe, but you're doing the right thing. The only thing. Sally's a young girl. People can take advantage of her in her current state. They might get the wrong idea. If she were my daughter I'd be giving her the exact same treatment." He moves toward the elevator, detaching himself from our despair—clinical, not cruel, an act of self-preservation. "Eventually the medication will start doing what it's supposed to do," he says, and rides back up to the ward.

Pat looks stricken, but steeled, fighting back tears. We agree not to leave. What if they decide to let us see her and we're not here?

We walk around the block to kill time. A nondescript street on the eastern edge of the Manhattan grid, indistinguishable from those around it. A woman enters a dry-cleaning store, presents the man behind the counter with a red ticket, and is handed a box wrapped with string, containing her blouse neatly folded perhaps, a laundered gift to herself, spotless and renewed.

When we return, nothing has changed. Visitors are leaving: the Hasidic family, the hipster. A few patients shuffle out for a smoke, the privileged ones, as I think of them, heavy-eyed, out of focus, like smudged photographs of themselves.

The nurse with the union pin comes down on her break, unexpectedly sympathetic now, as if we have passed some kind of preliminary trial. "Take it easy on yourselves, really, go home. You can always call. Just ask for Cynthia Phillips, I'll let you know how she's getting along."

Pat hands her Sally's night bag, a meager thing, yet for the time being our only point of contact.

"I'll see that she gets it. But you two go easy. You look like hell. She's going to need you, that girl."

Back at Bank Street I call Sally's mother and give her the news.

"No! You didn't put her away, Michael. You didn't!"

Put her away. The phrase has its impact. I remember it as a threat from childhood, usually directed at my brother Steve: We'll have to put you away. Do you want to be put away? Like some unwanted household object, I used to think, that for vague reasons of moral attachment can't be discarded outright.

"It's a hospital, Robin. There was no choice. She's very sick." I try to give her a sense of the past twenty-four hours, but how can I accurately convey the extent of Sally's transformation? Robin can't seem to follow me or fathom what I'm saying. And why should she? I wouldn't be able to fathom it either, our daughter suddenly out of reach, locked away with the severest cases, in some haunted place where we're not allowed.

I hear laughter in the background, Robin's husband good-naturedly scolding their dog. I imagine them sitting barefoot, on the back steps of their farmhouse.

"Michael, listen to me. Are you there?"

"Yes."

"Sally is having an experience, Michael, I'm sure of it, this isn't a sickness. She's a highly spiritual girl, I'm not the only one who says so, I have friends, psychically sensitive friends, who have met her and they say the same. One friend told me the heat radiating from Sally was more than she could bear. She never felt anything like it. And she's not a fake, Michael, I know what you're thinking, she's just a person like you or me with a gift for seeing what most of us can't. What's happening right now is a necessary phase in Sally's evolution, her journey toward a higher realm."

Her evolution. Her journey. I wanted to believe this too, in my way, when she was shivering with her *Sonnets*, awake all night. I wanted to believe in her breakthrough, her victory, the delayed efflorescence of her mind. But how does one tell the difference between Plato's "divine madness" and gibberish? between *enthousiasmos* (literally, to be inspired by a god) and lunacy? between the prophet and the "medically mad"?

Though I sense Robin wants to get off the phone, I prolong our conversation. "It's so beautiful here," she says, "so perfectly still. The mountains are like smoke. I'm starting to paint again." Her voice is like Sally's before all this began; their similar stops and inflections give me the odd feeling of being in contact with her. A momentary illusion.

I fall asleep on the couch, then wake up with a rush as if I've been shot from a cannon. I keep seeing Sally as a child, her tenacity, her warmth, her brushfire temper that I used to regard with exasperation—and sometimes with awe. Then the holding pen, the dungeon, where the maniac is restrained. Isolated behind a third locked door. Separated even from those who have been locked away from the world.

Pat wanders in from the bedroom, also unable to sleep. We sit together in the dark.

"Has she changed so completely or is it that I never knew her?" I wonder.

"You knew her," says Pat. "You still know her. She isn't gone."

I keep asking myself the obvious question, the helpless question. How did this happen? And why? One has cancer or

AIDS, but one *is* schizophrenic, one *is* manic-depressive, as if they were innate attributes of being, part of the human spectrum, no more curable than one's temperament or the color of one's eyes. How can something so inherent be a treatable disease? And how does one defeat such a disease without defeating oneself?

At 8:00 A.M., when the day shift comes on, I call Sally's ward. The woman who answers is guarded. When I ask for Cynthia Phillips, she says, "Cynthia's not available right now," and hangs up the phone.

At eleven we're at the hospital again, occupying the same plastic chairs. The guard gives no indication that he remembers who we are. At noon, however, he motions us over.

"You can go on up. Fifth floor."

Sally is transformed again, lying on her bed as if she's just been dropped from the sky, her hair splayed wildly around her. I sit down next to her, call her name. Minutes pass without a response. I call her again, touch her shoulder. She opens her eyes with great effort, lifts her head a few inches, and gives a gaping, slow-motion yawn.

"They think I'm crazy . . . did you tell them I'm crazy? Were you so afraid, Father, you told them to lock me up?"

She means to sound indignant but her voice is stifled and wobbly like a warped LP. Pat and I look at each other, stunned by the change. An immense apathy flows out of her. Her head falls back on the mattress. Her eyes close against her will, like dropped blinds.

"They stole my words," she says.

When we ask her what she means, she purses her lips and gives a sly, irritated laugh, a glimmer of her psychotic self that makes my stomach quail. Clearly she is in the throes of a second metamorphosis, every bit as violent as the one that brought her here. She sits up, the hectic glitter in her eyes wavering in and out of focus as if some battle for supremacy over her being were raging behind them.

I repeatedly try to break through to her, to establish some point of agreement between us (any point would do, an observation about the weather, or about the sky outside the gated window looming over her bed), each failure stabbing me as if for the first time.

Pat does better, but not by much. "Have you been sleeping, Sally?" she asks.

"I'm not sure," comes the delayed, foreign reply.

After a while, we both stop trying, the three of us sitting in the room like passengers in the compartment of a train. I hold her hand. "Sally, we're going to take care of you. You're going to be okay." She gives a muffled laugh that abruptly turns into a groan.

A nurse comes in to take her temperature and blood pressure. The room is so narrow that to make space for him Pat and I have to sidle over to the door.

"Ninety-eight-point-six," he says as the thermometer emits its little digital beeps. "Perfectly normal."

When he leaves, Pat decides to launch into action. From under the bed she retrieves the night bag we left with Nurse Phillips yesterday afternoon. It's obviously been searched. "They took the dental floss," Pat says. "And the lotion, probably because it was in a glass bottle. I should have known."

Sally's hospital gown is twisted around her, half the buttons unsnapped. The plan is to get her showered and into a pair of fresh pajamas. Pat coaxes her out of bed and leads her to the bathroom, shooing me out of the room.

Spilling into the hall from the room next door is the Hasidic family we saw in the lobby. There are at least eight of them, the women in long skirts, their shaved heads covered in ritualistic wigs and scarves, the men in *payess* or side curls and black hats. They're all eating from kosher plates they've brought, with the exception of the patient, their shoteh, who is poring over a black leather-bound Torah with a hollow intensity that reminds me of Sally with Shakespeare's *Sonnets*. His family surrounds him like a protecting herd: the curse of madness collectively borne by the tribe. Or so I imagine. I feel a surge of admiration and envy—for their solidarity, their numbers, their devotion to one another in the face of this bewildering storm. If only Pat and I could form such a phalanx around Sally! I nod to one of the men. He shoots me a sharp, disapproving look as if I've done something to harm him, and turns quickly, almost disgustedly, away.

Farther along the hall I come across the Quiet Room, easily identifiable even without the nameplate on its door. "Isolation." A tiny, fluorescent-lit cell, the walls padded with beige plastic foam, a single rubber-sheathed mattress on the floor. Shadowless, efficient, numbingly bland—a mockery of the Gothic chamber I had imagined.

A janitor is scrubbing what appear to be words off the floor, scrawled there apparently with a felt-tip marker. Nurse Phillips passes by, keys jangling. She smiles at me and continues on without pausing.

During the next few days I will piece together (from nurses, the attending psychiatrist, and in a fragmented way from Sally herself) what transpired after we left her in the ward that first night. Clutching the pen that the nurses had permitted her to have, Sally furiously began writing in her notebook. At the same time, the doctor ordered her first dose of haloperidol, a powerful neuroleptic widely used in the most acute cases of psychosis. Haloperidol is a descendant of chlorpromazine, the ur-drug of the psychopharmacological age. Its psychiatric value is its ability to induce indifference. ("The chemical lobotomy," psychiatrists called it when it was introduced in 1952, referring to the procedure that it rendered obsolete: the severing of nerve fibers in the brain's frontal lobes with a household ice pick inserted through the eye sockets.) And if excessive conviction, grandiosity, and fixed irrational ideas are among the symptoms of our most potent delusions, then indifference would seem to be a natural corrective, if not cure.

Indifference, however, isn't the only effect of these drugs—they also rupture much of the process of sequential thought. On chlorpromazine, the poet Robert Lowell was unable to build a three-letter word on a Scrabble board or follow the count of balls and strikes in a televised baseball game. Sally would experience a similar intellectual paralysis. Yet the drugs are necessary, the only way to wrench one from the grip of acute psychosis. In prescribing haloperidol for Sally, the doctor was responding to a medical emergency. Peter C. Whybrow, in his book, *A Mood Apart*, describes patients with "fulminating illness" like Sally's "who had dropped dead from manic exhaustion."

As it turns out, she was nearer to the abyss than we knew. Haloperidol blocks the production of dopamine, the neurotransmitter whose excessive presence in the brain was partly responsible (in purely chemical terms) for her distorted behavior. The brain's initial response to this blockade, however, was to produce more dopamine, faster (an attempt to compensate for the sudden stifling jolt), so that in a very short time Sally's mania shot higher, catapulting her to levels of psychosis she might never have reached without medication. She filled the pages of her notebook and continued writing— on the floor, the walls, the door. Thoughts rushed at her with unsustainable speed. But "thoughts" is the wrong word. They were more like explosions, as Sally would later describe them, visionary bursts in which the interconnectedness—the oneness—of the world was instantly revealed. The hospital became the place where genius is hospitably housed, the nurses the nurturers, the ward The Word . . . Zen Buddhists speak of satori, the rare instance when a novice is struck with the totality of the world in one. But what struck Sally was a kind of antisatori: her instant of epiphany shattered at once into chaos, only to reassemble and self-destruct again.

After crushing the tip of her pen, she ran out into the hall, her urge to impart, to enlighten, propelling her in every conceivable direction. She roused sleeping patients out of their beds, gripped them by the shoulders, led them staggering back into the hall. We are components of a single creative force, she tried to tell them, natural geniuses because this force is the embodiment of genius. When she opened her mouth to speak, however, what came out were not words, but a series of cracked, almost hesitant cries.

Responding to the disturbance, the night crew locked her in isolation, where she remained until the haloperidol successfully quashed the dopamine in her brain—a process that took about thirty hours.

When I return to the room Sally is freshly showered, wearing the silk fuchsia pajamas my mother gave her last month for her fifteenth birthday. Her head is on Pat's shoulder, her hair shiny and wet.

"I don't know who I am," she says.

"Did you ever know?" asks Pat.

She shakes her head, No.

"Then nothing's changed."

At 7:30 P.M. she is summoned by a nurse. Medication time. She gets up and walks into the hall. Another shock: two days ago she was coiled and lithe, wrestling Pat and me to a draw. Now she walks with a Parkinsonian shuffle, tentative and stiff. (A side effect of the haloperidol, I will learn; in *A Mood Apart*, Whybrow describes how dopamine helps drive the motor system and determines the fluidity with which we move our arms and legs. With her dopamine blocked, Sally's limbs have become like wood.)

She gets in line with the other patients in front of a booth where the meds are stored. A hushed decorum prevails; conversation, when it occurs, is conducted in a barely audible murmur. Along with Pat and me a few visitors are still hanging around. We give each other a wide berth, avoiding eye contact, tacitly agreeing not to pry. We have something in common that we're not eager to share. And what would we talk about if we were so inclined? There are no emblems of objective illness in the psych ward—no oxygen tanks or IV bags, no cardiac monitors or surgical wounds. Symptoms feel like intimate secrets; causes are elusive, cures unknown.

A dark, attractive woman in a wheelchair is in line in front of Sally. When her turn comes she stands without difficulty, swallows her meds, chats with the nurse. Gently, coaxingly, the nurse suggests she try walking to her room on her own. On hearing this, the woman's legs immediately turn to jelly and she slumps back into her wheelchair, her head in her hands in a gesture of sorrow so complete it seems to obey its own natural law.

Sally is handed her pills in a paper cup with ridges like a chef's hat. She takes them in front of the nurse and moves on.

"The halls are a maze," she says as we head back to her room. "Isn't that a-mazing?"

At eight o'clock we're politely told to leave; visiting hours are over. We ask Sally if there's anything she wants us to bring tomorrow. "Artichokes," she says. "And chocolate."

She climbs stiffly into bed, her mania wriggling under the surface like a cat in a zippered bag.

The Hasidim are in the lobby. To my surprise, the one who gave me a dirty look on the ward motions me over.

"What I'm about to say is not against your daughter. She's a friendly girl and I'm sure she means no harm. But she is disturbing my brother's peace of mind. In my religion, you see, contact with strange women is prohibited."

His brother's "peace of mind"? Has he forgotten where we

are? I don't like his reference to Sally as a "strange woman," as if she were tainted, a she-devil distracting his brother from his righteous path. Nor do I like his use of the term "my religion," excluding me from a practice that I too was brought up in, having spent eight years reading the five books of Moses in Hebrew as part of my daily diet in elementary school.

"How did she disturb him?"

She invaded his brother's room, he explains. She put her hands on him and forced him to look in her eyes. "She has no right to talk to him about what he believes. My brother is a gifted man. He has achieved *devaykah*," he adds cryptically, "the state of constant communion with God. Tell your daughter to leave him alone!"

"I'm sure the staff is equipped to handle these matters," I say curtly, and excuse myself, aware of his family watching us by the door.

On reflection, however, I understand where the Hasid is coming from: he has no choice but to believe his brother is holy; the biblical alternative is to be outcast from God. When Moses announced the penalties for disobeying God's laws, madness was first, before blindness and poverty, before the death of children, before war. Like the Hasid, I try to improvise my own area of protection around Sally. But I have little faith to draw from, either in medicine or God.

Putting his faith in the former, James Joyce took his daughter Lucia to an unending succession of doctors, certain that he would find her cure. One doctor gave her seawater to drink. Another ordered injections with a serum of bovine glands. In 1934 Joyce took her to see Carl Jung at his sanitarium near Zurich. To subject Lucia to psychoanalysis, concluded Jung, would be catastrophic. Successful analysis required the wounded sanity of the neurotic; it was useless in the face of psychosis. Instead, he was determined to analyze her father. Joyce's anima, or unconscious psyche, said Jung, was too identified with Lucia for him to accept that she was mad; to do so, thought Jung, would be for Joyce to admit that he himself was psychotic.

It was a questionable opinion, but it didn't contradict what Joyce himself had come to believe: that in some ineffable way he was responsible for Lucia's condition. Jung compared father and daughter to two people going to the bottom of a river, one falling, the other diving.

Yet the deeper Lucia fell, the more adamantly Joyce insisted that she was mentally sound—no madder, in fact, than he was. "Her mind is as clear and unsparing as lightning," he assured his son Giorgio. "She has the wisdom of the serpent and the innocence of the dove."

Joyce removed her from Jung's clinic and looked elsewhere for her cure. To no avail. Four years later he was telling Samuel Beckett that her mental distortions were caused by an infection in her teeth. "She's not a raving lunatic," he insisted, "just a poor child who tried to do too much, to understand too much."

I spend a fitful night on Bank Street, shuttling between dread for Sally's future and hope that somehow everything will be restored.

PART TWO

When Pat and I get to the hospital the next day, Robin is curled up with Sally, enveloping her on the narrow bed, the two of them apparently sleeping. Mother and child, a perfect tableau—mother six feet tall, willowy thin, pliant in a way that is immediately familiar to me. My first reaction is relief: the sight of them in each other's arms dispels the anxiety I'd been feeling about Robin's response to Sally in her current state. They appear to have slipped right into an unforeseen communion. Their slumberous breathing strikes a fairy-tale note of contentment.

"Like pals at a sleepover party," whispers Pat with a hint of resentment. She hesitates at the doorway, an involuntary flinch: the stepmother instantly overruled by Robin's biological assertion.

We fit ourselves into the tiny room and stand against the wall like the last two people in a lineup. The air-conditioning unit in the ward broke down in the middle of the night. Within minutes we are glossy with sweat. Beyond the gated window, the noonday sun in its haze looks like an egg laid by some giant bird. Below, the East River churns under the elevated road.

Their sleeping child
Among tygers wild.

When we were high school sweethearts, almost exactly Sally's age, Robin and I used to lie together in a similar manner, clutching each other for hours in her parents' apartment on Bleecker Street in Greenwich Village, sheltered in our adolescent cocoon.

Robin opens her eyes. "Michael, for heaven's sake, I didn't realize you were here." She peers drowsily at us from the bed, acknowledging Pat with a brief smile, meant to convey solidarity, I think, but falling short. "I jumped in my car at four this morning and drove straight through. Five hours. I couldn't stay away any longer, I had to see my daughter, *our* daughter, Michael, I was so afraid for her, I didn't know what to expect. After our telephone conversations, and the incident with the police and those horrible knives they had to hide . . . I thought she had changed shape or something. But just look at her, she's as beautiful and sweet as ever."

She indicates Sally, lying on the bed, not at rest so much as removed from consciousness, as if she was stopped in her tracks by a stun gun.

"She's on a great deal of medication," I explain, thinking of her scorched exaltations of a few days ago, the writing on the isolation room floor, the entire monstrous spectacle that Robin was spared.

Careful not to disturb Sally, she climbs off the bed and slips into her sandals. With Pat she goes out to the hall toward the dayroom, the large common area where patients and visitors pass the time. "I'll be right behind you," I say, remaining in Sally's room to do nothing more than listen to her breathing, and to ponder the undeniable mass of her on the bed and her shaken ephemeral fragility. A numbness comes over me that is like her numbness, I imagine, her knocked-out sleep, her distance from me and from herself—this hammered slumber that, I try to convince myself, is what will bring her back to me.

In the dayroom, Robin and Pat are making stabs at small talk. Pat invokes Sally's "willpower"; Robin predicts that she will emerge "renewed, stronger than ever." Joining them, I point out that tomorrow the holiday weekend will have ended, the staff will be operating at full tilt, and Sally will finally receive their full attention. "We may still find a simple explanation for what has happened. A trigger."

A man shuffles over to the snack table in the middle of the room, tears open a candy bar with his teeth and washes it down with fruit punch from a quart-sized tin can. Two patients argue over which video to insert in the VCR. A nurse named Rufus arrives, large-bodied and supremely bored. He confiscates the videos and switches on the television to a twenty-four-hour news channel: presidential candidate Bob Dole speedwalking down a Midwestern Main Street in a Fourth of July parade, flanked by screaming fire engines, marching bands, and grizzled contingents of other surviving veterans of the nation's wars.

Rufus mutes the sound, refusing eye contact with the patients. Like Nurse Phillips, he wears the union pin for local 1199 prominently on his uniform's lapel—Service Employees International, the definitive badge of his separateness from this place, of his independence, his distinction. *Your craziness can't get inside me*, it seems to be saying. *Now what about my pension?*

In a corner of the dayroom I spot the Hasidic patient, the shoteh, with his entourage. He looks more agitated than he did yesterday, his lips cracked and trembling, his eyes swollen with an indefatigable intensity. He clutches his black clothbound Torah on his knees and fiddles worriedly with the knotted fringes of his *tzitzis*—the garment that ultra-Orthodox Jews wear under their shirts as a spiritual version of a bulletproof vest. I am thrown back to my grandmother's kitchen as members of his family unpack their sanctified food: the aroma of kasha, barley soup, brisket of beef blending with the suety odor of the ward. Their shoteh sits pointedly apart, shunning them, praying in a feverish whisper. An older, stocky woman in a head scarf begs him to accept a plate of food. When he refuses, she places it under his chair and sits down beside him. His brother looks helpless and crushed. Catching my eye, he glowers at me with reinvigorated condemnation. I imagine the picture I must make with my two *shiksas*: Robin with her elongated Klimt-like figure and eggshell-blue eyes; Pat with her schoolboy haircut and balletic posture that must look to him like the very embodiment of pagan pride. His is a battle to multiply, to outlast, and hasten the return of the messiah. If he knew of my boyhood years studying Torah, he would despise me even more as an *apikoros*, the worst kind of traitor because I was brought up to believe and then willingly turned away from God.

To my surprise, Robin and Pat are huddled closely together now, in the midst of what appears to be an animated conversation, Robin's hand over Pat's in a gesture of fellowship, it seems—or is it to keep her from interrupting? We're closing ranks around Sally, I think, just like the Hasidim with their shoteh. We're a monolithic family unit, united in our concern for her, harmonious, getting along.

"Just look at what they're feeding her," Robin is saying, pointing to the snack table laden with packets of sugar and cupcakes. "Can you feel how wrong this is? I mean, how do you divorce a person's mental condition from her total organic well-being?" And to me, without skipping a beat: "This is exactly what *dis*-ease is, Michael. *Dis*-ease. How can anyone be *at* ease in this environment? Tell me."

I think: this is the sound of Robin's grief, her explanation for what none of us can comprehend. And I feel a rush of gratitude toward her for not pressing me for a detailed account of what led up to this. In Robin's shoes I would be demanding clues, facts, I would want to reconstruct every calibrated shift in Sally's behavior during my absence: When did she crack? When did she *almost* crack? What was the first sign? When did the eyes turn to polished coal and the words become incomprehensible? There had to be a critical instant, a turning point . . .

Pat, for her part, is attentive to Robin in the interested, appraising way of one watching a performance. Cheered by the apparent goodwill between them, I reach for Pat's hand. It slides away impatiently. She rises abruptly—"I have things to take care of"—and walks briskly out of the dayroom, to the nurse's station where Rufus is eating Chinese food in a take-out container and reading the *Daily News*.

By the time I excuse myself from Robin and go after her, Rufus has already let her out of the ward and relocked the doors.

SUPERMODEL MARGAUX HEMINGWAY TAKES OWN LIFE, reads the *Daily News* headline. "Was Reading Her Famous Grandfather's Books at Time of Suicide."

Sitting down again, Rufus tucks back into his meal. Politely, I ask him to open the doors for me as well. Aside from a barely audible sigh, he ignores the request, and I stand there waiting, holding my ground, until he rises in no particular hurry, his mystical thicket of keys dangling from the belt of his synthetic white nurse's pants.

I catch up with Pat as she is about to cross First Avenue with her tilting, slightly combative stride.

"Why did you cut out?"

"There's no reason for the three of us to cram ourselves into that room, staring at Sally like she's some specimen under glass."

"Robin could have warned us that she was coming," I say.

"I don't see why. She has every right to be here, more so than any of us. Why do you think they let her in before the start of visiting hours? They only do that for the mother, the sacred relation. Everyone understands this—except for you, apparently."

"What I understand is the awkward position you're in."

"That would surprise me, Michael."

A woman approaches and crankily demands a light for her cigarette. I'm almost certain I recognize her as one of the patients from the ward—on leave to wander the sweltering streets like the rest of us. Pat is kind to her; we have no matches. I want some of that kindness too. She says that she's heading downtown to her studio to catch up with work that might slip away if left unattended—classes and hourly renters that provide the cash to keep the studio alive. I detect a reproach in this. I should be working too, placing calls, shaking the trees for a new writing assignment. We mustn't allow things to fall apart. But I feel as if I've been struck with a kind of social amnesia, that my facility for casual conversation, for the necessary small talk that greases the wheel of reasonable cooperative exchange, has been lost.

"I canceled rehearsal," she says, referring to the piece she is in the midst of creating with her dance company for a show in the fall. They are scheduled to perform at a well-known theater in September, a booking Pat worked hard to obtain.

"I wish you hadn't."

"It's just as well. I've no idea what to do to the piece. Sally has managed to make the material I've been working on seem ridiculous. Suddenly it's beside the point, whatever the point may have been."

A picture comes to me of Pat in a solo dance I attended a couple of years ago, shortly after we met, when we were still sizing each other up, in the middle of a cautious mating dance of our own. It was the first time I saw her perform. *Monstrous Dragon* the piece was called, Pat reeling in a vest of tin cans, lit by car headlights at a club called The Gas Station on Avenue B on the Lower East Side. It was her aloneness in the white splash of those headlights that captured me, delicate yet unbreakable in her rattling dragon skin, with the power, it seemed, to evoke physical sensations that were transferable to the audience—or at least to me.

"Go back to the hospital," she says now. "You and Robin need to work this out together. It's from your life before me, I don't really have a place in it, and I'm not about to compete for one."

And with that she heads off toward the Lexington Avenue subway, in her signature walk—"ambivalent" was how I described it to myself the first time I saw it—self-regarding yet with an opposing wish to go unnoticed, to be left alone.

To be left alone. It was the first wish of Pat's that I absorbed when we met three years ago and our wariness of each other prohibited anything more than the careful cordiality that marked our unavoidable daily exchanges. We had been thrust together by chance when she moved into two tiny rooms at the back of the apartment on Bank Street. My old friend and landlord, seeking to earn a little more from the place, had installed her there, and I found myself having to compete with her for solo time in the kitchen, which we had no choice but to share. Pat would startle me with her silent catlike appearances at precisely the moment when I had assumed I was alone. She moved about on tiptoe—on dancer's point, I pictured her—with a self-effacement that seemed instinctive and refined. We conducted our territorial War of the Roommates in silence. Her shyness was practically a form of ostentation, and it seemed unlikely that we would manage even to strike up a friendship, much less become romantically involved.

Her existence was a paragon of simplicity: she seemed as free of material ties as she was of emotional ones, and devoted herself exclusively, as far as I could tell, to asceticism and art. Before leaving on tour with her dance company, she made me promise not to change the locks while she was away. When I expressed surprise—and annoyance—that she would think me capable of such an act, she said, without a hint of contrition, "It's ridiculous of me, I know. But worse things have happened."

What things? I wondered.

By the landlord's decree, I was to collect her rent and hand it over to him, which cast me in the unattractive role of her exploiter. She appeared to take pleasure in her position, and developed subtle ways of reminding me that morally she held the upper hand in our arrangement. It confirmed her pureness in her own eyes, I thought, and it was further proof of her stoicism, her regard for her life as some kind of ideal that she had to measure up to—irksome qualities, yet ones that despite myself I felt drawn to and admired.

More than anything else, her possessions were what fascinated me. Because they were so few they took on a charged air—her mother-of-pearl chopsticks, for instance, and her painted Chinatown bowl from which, after returning from marathon rehearsals of her dance company, she ate her late-night meals of tofu, angel hair spaghetti, and chard. More often than not she had to contend with a pile of dishes I'd left. She was a vegetarian, and my fried chickens and veal roasts were a philistine oppositional force.

One night, I caught her sliding her fingers through the drippings of a leg of lamb I had prepared. Bending forward so as not to stain her clothes, she sucked the crumbs of meat from her hand, blushing when she saw me, then withdrawing any hint of embarrassment as she grabbed her chopsticks and returned to her rooms in the back of the apartment, her chin shiny with pan grease.

The hypocrisy thrilled me. I decided that she was in the throes of a private war, with renunciation on one side and sensual pleasure on the other. I thought I saw evidence of it in her favorite garment, a coarse woolen sleeveless vest that sheathed her torso while baring her shoulders and long balletic arms; in the sternly hedonistic nights on the town to which she occasionally treated herself like a sailor on shore leave; in her impeccable yet vaguely self-mocking posture gained from years of Alexander Technique and martial arts; and in the torn green leather jacket that hung on her like a rag, pointedly unbeautiful, but with a certain ravaged glamour. With her ragged clothes and heavenward posture she gave off competing emanations of anarchy and control, elegance and disarray.

Her chief concern, and the one that eclipsed all others, was her dance company, for which she choreographed a series of gorgeous, enigmatic creations. Wyoming the company was

called, because of the sense of "emptiness" and "space beyond" that the word conjured. One of her heroes was Joseph
Beuys, whose "art actions" included locking himself in a New
York loft with a live coyote, a pile of hay, a felt blanket, and
old copies of the *Wall Street Journal*. "Beuys reconnected us to
what we are," she explained to me. "Flesh and blood. Violent.
Tame." Her dancers seemed literally to throw their bodies
away for no apparent reward other than the ecstasy of performing her work. One maxed out her credit card for the privilege of tumbling among the stones of the Trajan Market in
Rome (a site-specific performance). Pat, for her part, kicked in
most of her salary from her day job managing an off-Broadway
theater, as well as the modest grants she received, and spo-
radic donations from a handful of devoted fans. I admired this
sense of mission, but I was also a little wary. At its heart, I suspected, was a religious, possibly self-destructive hunger that
I had no hope of comprehending. I wondered if Pat, an Irish
Catholic by upbringing, was mistaking monasticism for art.

Austerity seemed to apply to her emotional life as well.
She seemed unsullied by intimacy, free of messy relations,
and this appeared to be a point of personal pride. She kept
everything streamlined, in check. With her dancers she was
intense, and strategically distant. Occasionally a lover climbed
the stairs to her room like a slotted visitor, departing after a
few hours.

Our first date was at the Metropolitan Museum to see the
paintings of the seventeenth-century Spanish artist Jusepe
de Ribera, in town on a visiting exhibition. An hour before
we were to meet, Pat phoned to cancel the date, then fifteen
minutes later called again begging me to forgive her for her

"foolishness" and announcing that our date was back on. We walked through the galleries, taking in Ribera's tenebrous assembly of martyrs on the cross. We came to a painting of Saint Bartholomew, wrinkled and naked, about to be flayed alive. "When I was seven a group of kids on the street tried to steal my hat," she said, laughing at the memory of herself. "I took off my overcoat and gave that to them too. I had just been taught the Sermon on the Mount and believed this was what I should do in the situation."

Now her life is entangled with mine, tainted by madness, and what is called for is a different kind of renunciation—one in which the rewards of self-expression are absent. I wonder if she is having second thoughts about our marriage, laden, as it is, with precisely the sort of distractions she had been avoiding before I came along. I want to tell her that Sally has reconnected us to what we are: *Flesh and blood. Violent. Tame.* Not from an "art action" but from the material core of her being, of her life.

But I'm not sure I believe it myself.

Rufus lets me rap on the door for a few minutes before admitting me back onto the ward. I get nowhere trying to engage him in a brief exchange—about the heat, the broken air-conditioning unit, the trials of summer. Big-bellied Rufus, Cerberus of the five-foot space between the elevator and the bolted ward, punishing me for having earlier interrupted his lunch.

Sally is in the manacled sleep that appears to have become her new way of being—the opposite of what she was just a week ago, which itself was a distortion of what she had been before. Robin is sitting at the foot of her bed, shut out from her just as I am shut out, but calmer than me, I think, with her enviable air of acceptance.

I half-expect her to accuse me of putting Sally here, of turning her into a *mental patient*, of betraying her in some fundamental way by robbing her of her epiphanies and branding her "vision" as insane. But she does not accuse, and gamely we endure our awkwardness with each other. We haven't spent so much time together since Sally's brother Aaron graduated from high school three years ago. Sally was there too, of course, twelve years old, proud of her brother yet overlooked at the table herself where we ate our celebratory meal and pretended for a day that our family was intact. She sat next to me with her head on my shoulder, enduring the meal, wishing for it to end.

"Have you spoken with Aaron?" Robin asks.

"Not yet."

"He's such a wonderful young man."

It feels oddly treasonous to be congratulating ourselves about Aaron in this way: our "bright spot," our trouble-free child, who has just completed his junior year at college and is currently away on a research trip for a summer fellowship he received.

"He's staying at a hotel," I say. "I don't have the number. I'm sure he'll call. It's strange to be out of contact with him. Especially now."

"I know."

With a shiver, Sally opens her eyes.

"Did you bring the artichokes, Father?"

"Artichokes?" asks Robin.

I explain that on leaving the hospital yesterday I had prom-ised Sally I would bring some, cooked, of course, along with a bar of chocolate, Sally's other wish. I didn't think the request was serious, and at any rate doubted that she would remem-ber. Another surprise. Maybe her memory now is keener than ever, imprinted with mania's branding iron.

I assure Sally that she'll have her artichokes tomorrow, but she gives no indication that she has heard me or cares.

"Tell me what I'm doing here," she says, puzzled and child-like, her eyes as black as obsidian, magnified and sharp.

"You're here to feel well again."

"I've never felt better. I'm perfectly fine."

"You haven't been acting fine."

"Everyone's acting, Father. You most of all."

"Sally, you're sick." I hear the flat insistence in my voice.

"*Sick. Mmm.* Does it make you feel safer to think of me that way?"

"We just want you to be yourself again."

"Your father doesn't mean that you're not yourself right now," says Robin. "He means, you're here, in the hospital to . . . *recover*."

Sally seizes the word. "Recover," she repeats. "But what have I lost? Or am I someone you want to cover up *again*. Some-one you want to put a lid on." Her voice hardens: the dreaded inquisitional tone. "You've always wanted to lock me up, Fa-ther. Now you've succeeded. You must be very satisfied with yourself."

She lets out a soft groan, then almost immediately bolts up from the bed as if yanked by a rope. Her arm shoots up at

74

an oblique angle from her body, where it freezes in what for all the world looks like a Nazi salute. Her neck is locked in an upward tilt too. She is standing by the window, unable to move, it seems, astonished by her predicament and by the startled look on our faces, unaware, it seems, of the bizarre statue she has become.

Robin lets out a quiet gasp, as I lead Sally back to the bed and sit her down. She tries to lower Sally's arm as if it were a pump handle, but it springs back up again to its permanent "*Heil!*"

Gently, I attempt to unlock her neck, but it too is fixed in this drastic tilt, like a mechanical toy. It looks unbearable, but Sally appears unperturbed.

"What have they done to her, Michael?"

Robin rushes out of the room and returns with Nurse Phillips, who casually slips her copy of *Jet* magazine into the pocket of her nurse's jumpsuit as she enters. "Black History Makers Honored at Gala Reception in Detroit," reads the cover.

"Feeling a little stiff, sweetheart?" she asks. She instructs Sally to "sit tight—no pun intended," and returns to the room a minute later with a syringe that she jabs into Sally's arm like an experienced cook tending to a pot that has boiled over: quick removal from the flame with no more than a flicker of annoyance.

"Cogentin," she informs us. "A muscle relaxant. Sally's a tad rigid right now. A side effect of her medication. It's completely normal."

"Shouldn't a doctor look at her?" asks Robin.

"That's unnecessary, dear. Believe me, this happens all the time."

Alone with Sally, Robin and I look at her as if she has been executed in front of our eyes. "They do everything but cure," I say of her myriad medications. The haloperidol has so thoroughly suppressed Sally's production of dopamine, the neurotransmitter that promotes quickness of wit and limb, that her body has entered a kind of rigor mortis. One phase of the war against mania has officially been won: a resounding victory over the riot in the frontal cortex of the brain's limbic system.

Less than five minutes after receiving the injection, Sally is able to straighten her neck and flex her arm. She flops across the bed in a melted state that is as excessive as the stiffness it has replaced. Only her hair, spread out in a tangled mass on the mattress, remains electrified and wild.

The day wears on with its out-of-time feeling, and we wait it out, Robin and I, pressed together in the cramped room, listening to Sally's shaken breath and her occasional oracular utterances.

"The curse of being beautiful is that we love ourselves too much," she says in her prophet's voice, waking for an instant and then falling asleep again.

We try to laugh; if only we could do so and mean it. An unexpected intimacy settles over us, the feeling that something has been restored: not our marriage, which we are relieved to be free of, or even our former affection for each other, but a flesh-and-blood rapport through Sally.

"It's hard to imagine New York isn't partly responsible for what has happened to her," she says. "The psychic strain here is enormous. Sally takes on the entire assault, the speed of the city, the toxins, she takes them in without filters."

"You always detested New York," I say. Although I wouldn't have guessed as much when I met her. Robin lived on Bleecker Street with her artistic-minded parents, and hung out at the Village coffeehouses, in perfect tune with the city, I thought, and, at fifteen, physically precocious enough to inspire the attention of older men who were a constant threat to me. She was majestically talented, as an oboist, a singer, and as a visual artist as well; she was a prodigy at the Art Students League. That her gifts were a source of distress to her perplexed me; she treated them as a burden she'd just as soon get off her back and discard.

The most meaningful events of her childhood, she claimed, were holidays at the Vermont cabin her parents bought as a getaway shortly after she was born. The cabin was upgraded year by year, so that its acquisition of electricity, plumbing, additional rooms, and new wood-burning stoves ran in step with Robin's own transformation from child to young woman. Vermont, she said, was where she came alive.

My attachment to the city was as powerful as her aversion to the place. She had pressed me to leave when Aaron was born, and then later, after we had Sally. But I couldn't conceive of living elsewhere. For ten years beginning in 1976, we resided on the border of Chinatown and the Lower East Side. Our nineteenth-floor apartment was level with the roadway of the Manhattan Bridge. Traffic ripped by our window on the bridge's steel grid. Below, on the East River, a prison barge was permanently moored; we used to watch the inmates play basketball, like miniature action figures, on its fenced roof each morning. Prostitutes serviced motorists in broad daylight under the elevated road. At night, gunshots between rival gangs interrupted our sleep. Trash smoldered in the empty lot across the way, and hovering above was a constant swarm of helicopters, monitoring traffic, going nowhere it seemed. The roar never ceased. For Robin our divorce was a repudiation of that roar, of the "Boschian underworld," as she called it, where I insisted on bringing up our children. It was a repudiation of her unhappiness, of New York, of me. She said that settling in Vermont—in a farmhouse located a few miles from her parents' place—was like breaking free of an extraneous predatory force. Sally too is a victim of that force, proving that Robin had it right all along.

Robin sits on the edge of the bed clutching her denim bag, from which she removes a half-ounce glass vial. "Skullcap," says the label, a flower extract and homeopathic remedy that, she shyly informs me, "promotes relaxation." The label is hand-painted in an Olde-Tyme apothecary style: a discreet corrective to the avalanche of medicalized concoctions from modern pharmaceutical labs. The herbalist in her forest hut, she measures a drop, gently opens Sally's mouth, and places it on her tongue as if feeding a rescued bird.

"I smuggled it in," she explains, pleased to have put one over on the staff. "They have a rule here against anything made of glass. You know, Michael, in the end, we're the only ones who can really take care of her."

She massages Sally's head, cupping it in her hands, finding the pressure points. Robin clamps her eyes shut to augment the intuitive quality of her touch. After a few minutes she moves to Sally's feet, pressing and palpating. She explains to me that it's a new therapy she has learned. "Polarity." It brings into balance the polar opposites of the body: the feet, which pound the grit of the earth; and the skull, the cranium, which points upward to that to which so many of us aspire— potentially sublime, but when cut loose from the earth, free-falling and lost.

"This is a particular area of concern for you, Michael, if you don't mind my saying so. You live so much in your head."

"I'm not as sold on my head as you may think."

"Well, you certainly used to be. I wasn't enough of an in-tellectual for you. I had the feeling I bored you."

"You never bored me. Not for a second."

"Only because you had no idea who I was."

Robin's New Age infatuations had been a bone of con-tention between us, and I can sense her bracing herself for some derisive comment such as I might have delivered during the disintegrating days of our marriage. She is going to make Sally well again. And why not? Her diagnosis seems as accu-rate as any: a psyche torn between its most extreme poles. What I marvel at is her physical ease with Sally. I have only one way to reach her: through language, the very faculty that has broken down.

"Mother dearest, are you trying to heal my heel?" says Sally, startling us from her far shore. "Or is your aim to de-feet me?"

This time we laugh together at Sally's punning, her hay-wire brilliance.

We remember Sally's birth, her head cocked improbably

high as if she was assessing the levels of energy in the room, her little nimbus of golden hair.

"I still haven't forgiven you for going out to eat while I was in labor," says Robin. "You were like that horrible Hemingway character who sits in a cafe with his ham and eggs while his wife is dying."

"The only reason I ate was so that I would have the stamina to stay with you when it counted."

"That wasn't the way it felt, Michael."

Watching them on the bed together now, I feel as if we are back in that birthing room, in a new version of her infancy.

"I felt a kind of electric shock when she was born," says Robin. "She was without stillness. She had no peace. She used to tremble and push me away with this enormous despair. There was nothing I could do to ease it." Robin's long emotive silences seemed to infuriate Sally. A voltage of discord ran between them. A month or two after she was born, she rejected Robin's breast, insisting on a violent autonomy. She seemed always to be waiting for some invisible storm to blow over. I sometimes worried that she felt at home nowhere, that what lay in store for her was a life in which she would be chasing one solution after another in a ceaselessly impulsive quest for some kind of haven from herself or just a place of pause. As a baby, lying on Robin's chest, Aaron had projected a bold and sturdy serenity. Sally had no such serenity. She was a thrasher, a gripper, a grasper, a yanker of fingers and ears. She thrust herself forward; she was relentlessly *propelled*. And unlike Aaron—with whom Robin's labor lasted twenty-six hours, Aaron resisting expulsion every inch of the way—she was born with supernatural ease. On first laying eyes on her,

I pictured a meteoric future. People instinctively gave way to her. She disobeyed. She bolted from Robin and me every chance that she had. Then, having contrived to make herself alone, she looked panicked and lost. She craved reassurance, but when we gave it to her she rejected it as tainted or insincere.

Now this second infancy, with Sally on the bed with her wayward black eyes, and Robin beside her administering her remedies and waging her healing campaign. As a baby, Sally wouldn't put up with this kind of communion with Robin. But now she offers no resistance. It is as if Robin is enacting with her the infancy she wishes they'd had.

I doze for a few minutes, and I am thrown back to when Robin and I were fifteen ourselves, hiding out in Robin's bedroom. It was almost as narrow as this one, and what comes back to me is Robin's luxurious silence, and the expression that accompanied that silence: at once tolerant and far away, an offering that also signaled her unconquerable detachment. I prattled on about my plans—our plans. And that expression of hers, that open-lipped half smile that encompassed to my teenage eyes the entire feminine world, was the only response I desired. We would lie together for hours, lost in each other, yet unaware of the other, with no danger of disagreement in our clutch, no room for potentially complicating intrusions.

I remind Robin of those Bleecker Street afternoons. "I still remember them as a kind of paradise," I say.

"Maybe for you it was. You've probably forgotten this, but

you used to tell me how 'liberated' you thought I was. I wasn't 'bogged down,' you said, by which you meant, I guess, that I was your idea of a free soul. You had no way of knowing this, but I was fed up with myself. I thought I was hopeless, everything I did felt stalled. My polarity teacher says I was stuck in shallow soil. Maybe that's why I understand what Sally's going through. She has nothing to hold on to, nothing to hold her down."

As if she is as startled by Robin's words as I am, Sally pops open her eyes, blinking us into focus, her face opening into a jubilant expression that immediately puts me on guard.

"Look at you two! I've brought you together again!"

Her smile is as broad as that of an opening night performer taking her curtain call, basking in applause. Another torn part of Sally's life has been repaired. The sheer power of her luminescence has brought Robin and me together again. All has turned out as she foresaw.

She orders Robin to sit next to me on the arm of the chair.

"Put your hand on his shoulder," she says. "Father, take Mother's other hand. Hold it tight."

When I hesitate, she glares at me. "Do as I say!"

Having arranged us to her satisfaction, she plants herself on the edge of the bed, hands clasped in her lap, enjoying the picture.

"You look beautiful together. Don't you realize this is the way you were born to be?"

7:55. Visiting hours are almost over. It is pouring rain, thick pellets slamming against the window.

I say good night to Sally, who is still aglow with the new harmony she believes she has imposed on our lives.

"Artichokes tomorrow," I promise.

"I'll stay a few minutes longer," says Robin.

We are off balance with each other after our mock re-marriage, and out in the hall we quickly arrange to visit Sally separately from now on, so as not to reinforce her false picture.

"The very idea that she believes there is some living ideal to go back to," whispers Robin.

As I am leaving, my attention is caught by a disturbance in the hall. Rufus is shooing the Hasidic family off the ward, rushing them into the elevator like evacuees.

The shoteh's brother gives me a stricken, possibly beseeching look as he is ushered away.

In the lobby he is wrapping his black hat in plastic, to protect it from the rain. His hands are trembling. He looks surprisingly fragile with his head uncovered, his hair above his side curls tousled and thin.

"They told us we stimulated him too much. It was an accusation. They marched him into his room like he was condemned."

"He'll feel better in the morning," I say.

It is still light outside, a yellowish twilight, enchanted in its way, with the thunderstorm pouring down, the raindrops as large as hailstones striking the ground like they've been hurled.

He seems to regret having confided in me, and turns abruptly away, leading his family, who are gathered around him, out into the storm.

Emerging from the subway at Twelfth Street and Seventh Avenue, I have the sense of having traveled from an alien place only to return to somewhere equally strange. The West Village has a stage-set feel. The thunderstorm has passed over but water continues to rush along the curb. The rain has darkened the pavement. The air is simmering. A drenched couple passes. The woman looks at her ruined shoes as if to say, Why fight it?

The 200-dollar hairdresser stands in front of his shop on the corner of Bank Street and West Fourth smoking a joint. He wears a red bow tie, leather suspenders, and, despite the heat, a striped Edwardian jacket. His powder-blue Vespa is parked on the sidewalk, glistening from the rain. "A heavenly weekend," he says to me. "*Tout le monde* has headed for the shore. We're socially disgraced, you and me. Positively marooned." Inside the shop, his implacable shih tzu lifts his leg over a mound of cut hair that has been swept into a corner.

Across the street is "my" building, like a derelict passenger on a first-class train. The bricks need repainting, the cornice is sagging, the lids have fallen off the beat-up trash cans. I climb the five flights to the campground of my apartment and collapse on the living room sofa. Sally's cracked Walkman sits on the steamer trunk that doubles as a coffee table, with Glenn Gould's Goldberg Variations still in the cassette slot. I try to turn it on. The batteries are dead.

Pat isn't home, and for the first time since he died two years ago I am overcome by a palpable desire to speak to my father. If only he were alive, with his horse sense and keen assessing eye. He was a hardnosed man, dealing scrap metal and pig iron from his warehouse in Brooklyn. Having had to contend with his own *shoteh* in my brother Steve, he would have understood the impact of Sally's crack-up. Of his own children, he used to say: "Whatever they are, I've no reason to act surprised." The fact that we were so often at odds only makes me miss him more sharply. When I was in my early twenties, with a baby to support, he offered me the chance to join him in the scrap metal trade. He was furious when I turned him down. "Those notebooks you scribble in won't get you on the goddamn subway," he said. Self-conscious about his lack of formal education, he took my literary pretensions as a personal affront. As a career, writing was unfathomable to him, unless you were as famous as Arthur Miller or cooking up gags for one of his revered television stars. Yet there is nobody with whom I could have spoken with less inhibition about Sally.

I nod off and then wake up with a start.

"You look like you just fell off a ladder," says the voice of my landlord Eric. He's standing over the couch, wearing work boots and a gray T-shirt torn around the collar. He's already helped himself to a bourbon. "I've been laying a new gas line. Honest work for a change. Is the fold-out bed still in working order? I'll be using it tonight, if you can put up with my snoring."

"I barely hear it."

He raises his glass as if to say *Salud!* Nothing is out of the ordinary; Eric crashes on the fold-out when he pleases, at least four or five nights a month.

Reaching into his shoulder bag, he removes a manuscript copy of the novel he has been working on for years. "I've completely revised it," he says. "Would you mind having a look?

Some of the changes are subtle, but taken as a whole I think they make a real difference."

One hundred and fifty-eight pages, I notice, the same length as when he first showed it to me shortly after I moved in. Perhaps my encouraging words at the time were influenced by my dependence on him. But there were things to admire in his writing—a certain wryness, a curious feeling for people with power. About a year later, after a much talked-about "rewrite," he gave me the manuscript again. As far as I could tell, not a word had been changed. I pointed this out to him as gently as I could. "You're right," he said. "I need to get on with it, take the bull by the horns!"

Since then, I've gone out of my way to avoid the subject, but Eric constantly brings it up, counting on me to endorse his illusion by discussing the novel in such a way as to make it seem viable and alive. I've come to realize he has no more intention of finishing the novel than of abandoning it. He speaks of it the way one speaks of moving to Tahiti or sailing around the world. Yet I can see that on some level it causes him pain.

I gather up the manuscript and place it neatly on my lap. A tacit promise. I feel as if I'm impersonating the person I was before Sally's crack-up. If Sally had been in an accident or come down with some overtly physical disease, I would not hesitate to tell him about it, confident that his sympathies would flow in my direction as a matter of course. But psychosis defies empathy; few people who have not experienced it up close buy the idea of a *behavioral disease*. It has the ring of an excuse, a license for self-absorption on the most extreme scale. It suggests that one chooses madness and not the other way around. When Eric refers to someone as "crazy," he means uninhibited, rebellious, creative. It's a form of praise.

"Does Pat have a problem with me?" he suddenly asks.

"Of course not."

"She called earlier. She seemed . . . put out. Impatient. And not for the first time. It's a general feeling with her. How shall I put this? I don't feel *welcome* anymore when I come around."

In my own place, he might have added. Our leap, Pat's and mine, from obscurely hostile roommates to married couple has radically altered the chemistry of my friendship with Eric. Pat is unwilling to play along with the crash pad atmosphere Eric and I maintained before she came on the scene. Eric misses our bachelor days.

"I'm going to visit some friends uptown," he says frostily. And he abruptly leaves.

10:25. I replace the burnt-out fuses and switch on the air conditioner, which then labors away like an old truck in the corner. Eric forgot his newspaper, the front page of which informs me that Vicente Gigante, the most powerful mafia boss in the United States, is wandering around Greenwich Village in his bathrobe and slippers, hollow-eyed, unshaven, pretending to be insane so as to avoid having to stand trial for murder. "He's a scary person," says a neighbor. "He stares right through you like you're not there."

A parody of madness. What other disease is verifiable solely from the social affect of its victim?

On another page of the paper more news of Margaux Hemingway, dead at forty-one from an overdose of barbiturates.

Her grandfather had also killed himself in the month of July, thirty-five years ago, with a shotgun. He had been trying to perform the opposite trick from Gigante's: that of convincing people that he was sane so he would be left alone long enough to put an end to himself. He was taken to the psychiatric section of the Mayo Clinic in Rochester, Minnesota, after a gun aimed at his face was wrested from his hands. At the Mayo Clinic he "charmed and deceived [the doctor] to the conclusion that he was sane," wrote his widow Mary.

The phone clatters to life. "Pops!" It's Aaron, his voice infused with a delight that I immediately find myself clutching at while trying to conceal the weight in mine. He's calling from a motel in Youngstown, Ohio, where, for his fellowship, he is studying the economic depression that has befallen the city since its steel mill shut down.

"I had lunch with the mayor. The *mayor*, Pops. He couldn't wait to see me. It's the same with everyone here—they want to talk, they *need* to talk, partly because they have so much time."

He describes the city, people wandering the streets day and night, in a hell of idleness. Like on the psych ward, I think. But I don't say so. I'm too busy soaking up the lifeline of his voice, the casual nature of his closeness to me, his observations, his engagement. His sanity.

After we've talked for several minutes, I still haven't told him about Sally. Why cast a pall over his excitement? He can't do anything to help her right now; he'll find out soon enough . . .

"How's the motel?" I ask.

"It's another casualty of the steel mill. I'm the only guest. It used to be a Ramada Inn. A Bangladeshi family owns it now. They're closing down at the end of the month."

As soon as our conversation ends, I realize the mistake I have made: Aaron won't feel "protected" from the news I've withheld, he'll feel lied to and fooled. *You let me chatter about Youngstown while my sister was being declared insane?* How would I explain to him that I had been protecting myself from having to relive the shock of Sally's crack-up through her brother's eyes?

I have turned out the lights so as not to overburden the wiring while the air conditioner is on, and the apartment is lit solely from the street: the tall halogen lampposts below and the pale lunar blueness seeping down from Times Square.

It's after one o'clock when Pat comes home.

"I fell asleep," she explains. "In the studio. We've been hit by a hammer, Michael."

"Did you get any work done?"

"I managed to persuade two dancers to show up on short notice. I had no idea what I was doing. If the dancers could tell, they were polite enough not to let on. How's Sally?"

I fill her in on the day's events: Sally's sudden stiffness, and her belief, on waking, that she had brought Robin and me back together.

"That's what she really wants. The three of you together. It's why I left you alone."

"We've decided to visit her separately from now on."

"That's entirely your call. Like everything else about this."

"I'm sorry."

"I don't see why. I'm not angry with you, Michael."

She looks exhausted and unusually pale.

"I called earlier to see if you were home. Eric answered. He didn't sound overjoyed to hear my voice. I asked him if any messages had come in. I was thinking of Sally. I wanted to know if she called—what a hopeful sign it would be if she had! Or if you called with news. Eric acted like I was asking him for a loan. He doesn't like me."

"You didn't tell him about Sally, I hope."

"Of course not."

"I wouldn't want him to know about her. It's not that I'm ashamed of what's happened. But he wouldn't understand."

"No one understands. *We* don't understand."

"He'd tell our friends. It would make life more difficult for her. People would start thinking of her as weird. Stained."

I wake before five, Pat lying next to me on her side, Eric snoring on the fold-out bed in the living room.

I tiptoe out of the apartment, carrying my shoes and putting them on in the hall. At a twenty-four-hour vegetable stand on Greenwich Avenue, I buy artichokes and a bar of dark chocolate, then kill time walking the streets while daylight seeps into the city like smoke and the coffee bar on Eighth Avenue opens, and a few people straggle out of their buildings searching for cabs.

Later, I steam the artichokes and wrap them in tinfoil for Sally.

The moment I enter the hospital lobby, the *shoteh*'s brother rushes over as if he has been waiting for me to come through the door. I brace myself for a fresh barrage of complaints about Sally, but he surprises me by thrusting out his hand and introducing himself by name: Yankel.

"They're telling me that Noah is in the Quiet Room," he says, referring to his brother. "They won't let us up to see him. Not me, not even his mother. Like we are the cause of Noah's *tsorres*. This 'Quiet Room,' you know what it is?"

I hear myself trying to describe it in benign terms, without believing them myself.

Yankel interrupts me.

"What do they know from 'mental illness' in this place? Maybe you can explain to me what such an expression means. I took Noah to the rebbe who said that he has become lost in his pleading to God. 'I can't help you with this,' he told me. 'Go see a psychiatrist.' Our own rebbe! He should know better. There is no medicine for this. Not for Noah or for your daughter either."

Sitting a few feet away in a plastic eggcup chair is the stout babushka woman whom I've noticed before: Noah and Yankel's mother. Next to her is the madman's bride, ripely pregnant and no older than eighteen. She seems timid and bewildered, her wig a luminous bundle of black human hair, shorn from the head of a woman in India, no doubt, Hindu hair being the Orthodox wigmaker's main source of supply.

The mother begins to cry. Yankel ignores her but looks on the point of tears himself. The girl stares determinedly at her hands in her lap.

"Maybe this was our own doing," says Yankel. "We encouraged Noah to be aloof because he had such a gift. You know what means 'aloof'? Existing in the spirit world, the higher realms. When he was fifteen he went through the entire cycle of the Talmud in a single year. Five thousand pages.

The most revered scholars take seven years to do this. People think he's *meshugah*. But this is not the case. I'm not ashamed to tell you, he talks directly with his phantoms. There was a time when I believed it was the Creator he was speaking to. And I'm still not convinced it isn't so."

He looks to his mother for encouragement, her legs crossed at the ankles, her stockings sagging slightly, her feet clad in slablike orthopedic shoes.

"He sees what other people don't see," he continues, "including some in our own community, God protect them, I won't mention any names. They've been taught the mysteries but they haven't comprehended them like Noah. Now they'll brand him a *hefker*. You know what is a hefker? An animal. A person outside the fold."

"Chances are he won't be in the Quiet Room for long," I say. "In fact, it may actually protect him."

"You think my brother needs protection *from himself*? Does it occur to you that Noah is alone in a sea of bliss while the rest of us are mere islands of misery?" He pauses, softening his voice with visible effort. "Noah's problem is that he is not acquainted with the mundane. 'When you feel ripped from the ground go build something,' says the wise man. 'Work with wood. Lay brick and mortar. Get on your hands and knees and scrub the floor.' When Moses sent spies to scout the Promised Land, some of them didn't like what they found. They preferred life in the desert, with its miracles and manna from heaven, where they could meditate and live free. They didn't want to enter the land 'that consumes its inhabitants,' as the psalm says. The land with all its troubles, God help us. But one must enter the land. The land is where life is."

He clasps my arm, moving us out of earshot of the women. "Will you check on him when you go upstairs? I'll wait for you down here. You'd be performing a mitzvah. I just want to know he's okay."

I have to stand on my toes in order to look through the netted glass slit near the top of the Quiet Room door. Noah is sitting just as Sally must have sat, cross-legged on the rubber mattress. He is rocking back and forth—the hypnotic davening of the Hasidim—in what appears to be a state of ecstatic prayer. His yarmulke has fallen off and lies inside out, its stitching showing, drained of significance. The fluorescent ceiling light burns in its flat, saturating way. Noah's prayer book is in shreds, its pages strewn on the floor. His *payess* have lost their buoyant twist. I am struck by his bare feet, his awkward boyish beauty, long-limbed and oddly refined. He looks nothing like his brother. He is nineteen, Yankel told me, four years older than Sally. A paper cup filled with water is by his side. In a delicate choreographed manner, he dips his fingertips into the cup and rubs the water on his eyelids with their faint blue veins. He seems to relish his solitude, conversing without interruption with his living God, like Elijah in his cave talking to the birds. I try to imagine Sally in this room, writing as fast as she could on the floor with the felt-tip pen that the nurses had permitted her to have, bending their own rules, I now realize, taking a chance that she would not swallow it or use it to poke out her eyes. What inner crumble must she have experienced, with her terrified grandiosity, throwing herself against the beige walls. "What purpose is there in madness?" King David asked God after he had gone incognito about the city and beheld the mad among the crowds in the marketplace. "When a man goes about and rends his garments, and children mock him—is this beautiful in Thine eyes?"

"This isn't a sideshow, Mr. Greenberg."

Cynthia Phillips has caught me with my face pressed to the glass.

"I'm on a mission for Yankel," I explain. "Is it common for a patient to be in isolation after an entire week on the ward?"

"I'm told Noah was shouting at your daughter last night, but I wasn't here."

I go to Sally's room. She's on her bed, out cold. I set the artichoke on her bedside table, with a plastic container filled with lemon and olive oil dressing, Sally's favorite. I'll have to make a special plea to Nurse Phillips for a knife sharper than the plastic ones to cut out its heart.

I brush a mutinous lock of hair from Sally's cheek and lightly shake her arm.

"I brought you an artichoke."

"Art makes you choke, Father. You should give it up. It's a false god who causes you nothing but pain."

Another oracular pronouncement. Blinking at me, she emits one of her mighty yawns, then slips back into the River Lethe. The nurses have assured me that this lethargy is merely a phase, but no one will venture to say how long it is expected to last.

Rufus lets me off the ward with a curt nod, and I take the elevator back down to the lobby where Yankel is waiting, anxious for news.

"When will they let us see him?"

"Probably tomorrow. When Sally was in isolation we were able to visit her the next day. Other than that, I've nothing to go on."

"You think I do?"

"He isn't suffering," I say, though I have no way of knowing this for certain. "He looked well."

I glance at his mother and young sister-in-law, sitting where I left them in their broiling wigs and ankle-length Orthodox garb. The girl assiduously avoids my eyes, looking like a child in a dentist's chair.

"Did he have his prayer book?" asks Yankel.

"Yes."

"Idiots! They think they're doing him a favor by letting him have it, they're being sensitive to his *special cultural needs*. They understand nothing. Heaven knows what sin he'll bring down on himself with that book. I should have taken it from him myself. I only pray that the One Above isn't paying attention."

"If He *is* paying attention, we can assume that He understands the situation perfectly. Since He created it Himself."

"He *is* attention," says Yankel stiffly.

"Have you been married long?" I ask the girl.

"Eight months." Yankel's mother answers for her. "Noah never raised a hand against her. There will be no divorce unless he decides to grant one. And as long as he is in no condition to decide such a thing, they will remain wed. The rebbe knows this perfectly well. It's the law."

The girl maintains her bewildered silence, either unable to speak or prohibited from doing so. She is saddled with a husband whose devoutness was probably presented to her family as an asset when the marriage was arranged.

She watches her fidgeting hands as if they were two small pets in her lap.

The following afternoon, Sally and Noah are ensconced in the dayroom talking intensely. Noah seems transfixed by her. His feet are still bare, his Quiet Room joyousness undiminished.

"They have a way of finding each other," says Yankel, resigned, it seems, to the effect on Noah of Sally's she-devil allure. Noah's prayer book is gone; I hope Yankel didn't see what he did to it.

"Do you find that you can't sleep?" he asks. "I keep Noah in my head. I try to make the best of it. If only I knew the song young David played to soothe Saul."

"It didn't soothe him for long," I say.

"All I ask for is the miracle of a few hours."

Yankel watches his brother closely, but when Noah looks in his direction, he quickly drops his eyes, wary of setting off a fresh spark, perhaps, or too stricken to engage him.

At six o'clock Yankel announces that he must leave. Every Thursday he delivers food to the homes of the poorer members of his sect in Brooklyn. "We all chip in. They would do the same for me, heaven forbid I should need it." The vans are disguised as commercial delivery trucks with the names of actual grocery stores on them. "So no one is humiliated. No one feels singled out for having less."

The aim is to hasten the appearance of the messiah on earth, an event that requires a measurable accretion of mitzvahs or righteous deeds. After enough mitzvahs have been performed, the cosmic scale will tip to the side of God, and humanity will be bathed in holy goodness.

One such mitzvah would be to persuade me, a lapsed Jew, to pray with him. With this in mind, he removes a set of tefillin from his pocket: the black cubes containing minutely copied passages of Scripture that devout Jews fasten to themselves by means of a complicated array of leather straps. Would I allow him to tie me up in them? I decline politely. "It would be wasted on me. I'm sorry." And right there, in the dayroom of the psychiatric ward, Yankel Mandelbaum proceeds to wind the leather straps around his own left arm and fingers while muttering a Hebrew prayer.

Spotting him in the midst of this ritual, Rufus demands that Yankel put the tefillin away at once. "My patients could strangle themselves with that contraption!"

Yankel rises to leave, dripping with sweat, "May you sleep like a baby tonight, Noah," he says. "You and me both."

The dayroom door opens and Pat arrives from dance rehearsal, vibrant and spent.

"I've shifted gears completely," she says of her dance-in-progress. "It's a different piece."

Sally and Noah huddle even closer. Noah disappears under his prayer shawl like a ghost in a sheet. Sally says that he is "inside a cloud." Noah prays in a lisping voice that resembles soft giggling. Sally yanks the prayer shawl from his head. Noah calls her a "demon." Rufus comes over barking, and steers them apart.

Pat and I escort Sally to the opposite side of the dayroom. She spins around, seizes my arms, shivering through gritted teeth and shaking me violently. I have thwarted her again! I am the one who stands in the way, the one who douses the flames of her visions and prevents them from lighting the world.

A tall, striking woman with cascading gray-blond hair commands Sally to release me: Dr. Elizabeth Mason, I read on her name tag. She caught sight of Sally's little meltdown as she was passing along the hall. "We do not touch people here. We keep our hands to ourselves!" She towers over Sally and has to bend down to look her squarely in the eyes, her voice briefly crossing over to a manic cry of its own. "We have already discussed this, Sally. *Hands to ourselves!*"

Sally obediently backs off.

"She means no harm," I say.

"Here we have a different definition of 'harm.'"

I introduce myself as Sally's father.

"I gathered as much. On this ward we respect one another's personal space. I've no doubt you can see the wisdom in this."

Sally shrugs as if to say, *What can I do? This is the way they are.*

"While she's here, your daughter will be under my care. We've already had a few interesting conversations, haven't we, Sally?"

A timid nod of the head in response.

"I can assure you that she is as shocked by what has happened to her as you are. We'll schedule a family meeting at some point. I have your number. Expect a call."

With that, she heads off toward the staff room: a command post enclosed in glass where a scene of muted busyness is played out among phones, computers, diagnostic manuals, drug promotions, medication schedules, and charts—a visible contrast to the aimless activity of the rest of the ward. It promises us that there is a higher intelligence at work. A strategy. A grand plan.

Pat and I escort Sally back to her room.

"She never learned to respect boundaries," says Pat. "You and Robin weren't able to teach her that."

"Maybe you should discuss it with the staff," I snap.

"Oh, I think they know all about it already."

Later, I spot Noah praying at maximum speed, his lisping voice growing louder. The next day he is moved to a different ward.

Robin phones from her aunt's apartment on Bethune Street to inform me that she must return to Vermont. "George is running the bakery alone. It's too much for him. I hate to leave Sally, but my husband needs me too. I miss my home, Michael." She pauses. "I just don't feel like I can do anything for her while she's behind those locked doors. She sleeps and sleeps. Like she's reassembling herself in some way, with or without me. I would stay if I thought it would help her even the tiniest bit."

"I know."

"Maybe what we need to do right now is give up the idea that we can save her."

We meet at a health food store near the hospital after she has paid her good-bye visit to Sally. Robin is at the end of her rope. The dis-ease of New York has caught up with her, she tells me. "I stepped on a dead pigeon. I feel utterly nauseous."

I walk her to her car. It's an infernal afternoon. Robin presses a handkerchief to her face, as if we are walking among corpses: the charnel breath of July in New York. A street-cleaning truck wobbles past, its scrub brush spinning along the curb, sending scraps of garbage flying.

"I'm glad the three of us could spend a few hours together," she says. "To be honest, I was nervous about seeing you. But we did okay. I wish I could explain what has happened to Sally, even if it means blaming myself or us. I wish we could say, 'It was pesticides or a vaccine or something she ate . . .'"

She unlocks her Honda. A small wooden bear with a flowing back and bemused expression hangs from the rearview mirror: one of Robin's exquisitely wrought carvings.

"I've learned to make these things without expectations," she says in response to my appreciative comment. "It only took me twenty-five years to stop caring about whether people think it's art."

She pulls out of her parking space, then stops and rolls down the window. "I'm choosing to be optimistic. I refuse to see this as an ending for Sally. Her thoughts are just traps, you know."

"I'll call you at the slightest development," I say.

"I know you will. I'm trusting you, Michael."

She drives away.

Keep your empathies to yourself. Avoid eye contact with patients. Never argue. Resist overidentifying with others, and maintain the illusion of privacy with fellow visitors as you would with picnickers on separate blankets in a crowded park. Make friends with members of the staff, if possible, and expect nothing in the way of reassurance from them in return.

After seven or eight days, Pat and I have become old hands on the psych ward, initiates to its tacit code of behavior and arcane ways. The guard in the lobby who barred our entrance when Sally was in isolation nods cordially at us now; and upstairs, Rufus unlocks the door for us as a matter of course. We have slipped into the rhythm of the place, becoming familiar with patients and staff the way one becomes familiar with faces on a commuter train.

Pat makes no comment on Robin's departure. "The real mother," she calls her. She is as dutiful with Sally as ever, holding her in the clear pool of her attention. She listens to her with eyes half-closed. Sally, in turn, treats Pat as if she alone understands the spectacular workings of her mind. "I'm wired for this. It's automatic," says Pat with a certain soldierly aplomb.

We try to be gentle with each other, but the strain shows. "Do you think she'll snap out of it?" I ask one too many times.

Pat's neutral answer disheartens me. Unreasonably, I want her to be more certain. Occasionally she jots something down in her notebook. "For my piece," she explains.

"Are you finding material in all this?" I ask with a hint of annoyance.

"I don't look at it that way," she says, and disappears to phone her dancers, to set up another rehearsal.

The days pass. We are a silent force in Sally's room. I tell myself that a kind of stasis has been struck. Sally has not grown worse, she is in abeyance, safely confined in a "holding environment," as the psychologist Donald Winnicott called it.

Watching her in the straitjacket of her medication, I sometimes can't tell if she is awake, and wonder if the two states are indistinguishable to her as well. She is in no-man's-land, I think, what the Buddhists call *bardo*, the state between the death of one incarnation and the birth of the next, where the "disembodied mind" hovers, neither here nor on the other side.

A rare breeze passes through the room, and Sally says that the air is "tickling" her like "a feather." Her languor lifts, and then returns with its downward tow. She digs her fists in her eyes, smiles apropos of nothing, and then treats me to a fresh vituperative burst. Just when her mania appears to be definitively routed, it mounts a new potent charge. At such moments she seems to be clinging to it as to her very being. I imagine the mania as a separate living thing within her, a gnome, like Rumpelstiltskin, wily and insistent. It speaks to her in a whisper, promising riches, deviously finding a way to escalate and live on.

I decide to bring her something to read. Books are out of the question: they would only drive home the fact that her concentration is shot. A magazine would be more suitable, I think. But which to choose? The one about celebrities is too grandiose; and the magazine about the travails and glories of being a woman seems cruel with its promotion of a perfection beyond Sally's grasp. I settle on one devoted to food, and place it on her bedside table. Sitting there, its cover, which reads "Eleven Things You Can Do With Blueberries," looks absurd.

While Sally sleeps, I pass my time in the dayroom, sitting in my favorite spot under the reproduction of a painting by

Chagall: a couple on a wooden bench, a picket fence in the foreground, and a shabby angel hovering over them under a full moon. Patients trickle in and out of the room, looking like photographs that didn't quite get developed in the lab. It is the ward's public square. A dark-haired woman enters in a wheelchair, pushed by a young rail-thin man in a Panama hat and white linen jacket. I recognize her from the medication line. On her lap are a blue cashmere throw and a small pile of books: *Darkness Visible*; *The Bell Jar*; *An Unquiet Mind*; *Girl, Interrupted*—the contemporary texts of mental disturbance. They park themselves in a corner, with the air of aristocrats who have been exiled to some backwater town. The man caresses her hand, maybe to reassure her. With a folded handkerchief he lightly pats the sweat on her forehead.

The following day I catch sight of her in the hall, demanding that Nurse Phillips push her into the dayroom. "You can perfectly well get up and walk there on your own, Kara," says Phillips, as if talking to a child. Furious, Kara propels herself down the hall, hand-powering the wheels like one who has been forced into the indignity of menial labor. I enter the dayroom behind her and sit down under the Chagall. The television is blaring. A visitor pores over the horoscopes in last week's *New York Post*. After glancing about the room, Kara parks herself next to me. "They've put me on some kind of suicide watch," she says as if making small talk that bores her. "It's totally ridiculous. There's nothing wrong with me that a competent neurologist couldn't get to the bottom of, if such a person exists in this godforsaken place."

Shielding her eyes from the sun, she looks out of the padlocked window at the stacked towers of the East Side.

"I blacked out, and when I came to I couldn't move my legs. As soon as my father comes, he'll get me a real doctor and all this nonsense will be finished. He promised he'd come."

She acidly calls the psychiatrists "those superintendents of sanity," discounting their medical expertise and demoting them to custodial status. Indicating one of the patients, she declares: "They've given her the wrong medication." Of another, she says, "They don't care what's really going on inside him. It's all about symptoms. Zero emotion."

Agreeing, I mention a paradox of psychiatry: mental illness is recognized by the patient's distorted thoughts, but treatment is largely indifferent to their content. "You're just like the rest of them," Kara says, and she brusquely wheels herself to the opposite side of the dayroom.

In her room, Sally wakes up and flips through the magazine I brought. "Yum. Blueberries." I laugh, gratified, as she studies the glossy pictures. On my way out, I spot the young man with the Panama hat, finishing his own visit. Kara rises from her wheelchair and walks him to the door. She doesn't seem to realize that she is on her feet, until Nurse Phillips, about to unlock the ward's main entrance for him, says, "Maybe it's time we put away the cripple's chair." As if on cue, Kara begins to teeter. With a hint of impatience, Phillips grips her arm before she topples over.

"Come on, sweetheart. You're not going to get what you're after by pretending you can't walk."

With Phillips's assistance, Kara limps back to her room like an injured athlete.

The next day, she wobbles fawnlike into the dayroom on her own, clutching a notebook with a pen jammed in its spiral binding. A triumph. Her mother is waiting for her, along with the young man with the Panama hat, who, I now realize, is her brother. He seems more captivated than ever by her strict beauty: her cracked lips and fair skin and burnished raven hair. In a bright bristling voice, her mother describes an art exhibition she saw earlier in the day. "Wonderful work, by a woman no older than you, Kara. Disturbing, but in a positive way."

Kara announces that she feels chilled. She rises to go to her room, but her legs buckle under her and she flops back into her seat. Her brother tries to help her up, but she pulls away from him. I have the irrational urge to stand in for her father, who has failed to show up. I could do for her what I have been unable to do for Sally. But what would that mean? Catching my eye, Kara turns away with majestic apathy, and then buries her head in her hands.

When I learn that she has been discharged, I ask Phillips if she was able to leave the ward walking.

"I can't tell you that, Mr. Greenberg," she says. "You should know better than to ask."

In the morning, Aaron phones me from Ohio. "I feel like I'm in one of those scorched-earth movies about the future. Everything decent has been destroyed. You realize how powerless we are in the face of some asshole's decision to turn a quick profit simply because he can."

He is at the airport, on his way back to college in upstate New York.

This time I try to give it to him straight. I hear the words "crack-up" and "hospital" come from my mouth, and realize that he thinks I am describing an accident involving a car.

"No, no, the crack-up was in Sally's head," I say. "It happened from one day to the next. I don't know how to describe it. She just fell away."

"I don't get it."

"She's in a psychiatric hospital."

I sense him scrabbling to get a handle on this. "Are you telling me my sister is insane? Who decides such a thing? I don't even know what the fuck it means!"

"No one decides. It's not a decision."

"This is such bullshit."

"I keep hoping that's the case."

"Is Mom there?"

"She was. She had to go back to Vermont."

"Did you think I couldn't take it, Pops?" He has figured out that I kept the truth from him when he phoned a couple of days ago from his motel in Youngstown. "You could have let me help you."

Pat is sitting at the dining room table writing in her notebook. I read over her shoulder: *The voices inside the dancers' heads. Whispering to them from behind. Relentless.*

"Aaron, what you're doing is important. I don't want this to stop your life the way it has stopped mine."

"I'm changing my flight," he says. "I'll see you in a couple of hours."

He arrives at the hospital late in the afternoon, six feet two, round-faced, handsome, bursting into Sally's room with his playful rolling stride.

"Scooch, you look fantastic," he says, using his pet name for her. "What are you doing in this place?"

He comes laden with presents—the *New Yorker*, *Newsweek*, *People*, *Vogue*—the very magazines I had pondered over and decided not to bring.

"Did Father tell you why he locked me up?"

Aaron envelops her in his arms, loving and offhand, hiding his distress.

He beckons me out into the hall. He looks thinner than the last time I saw him, and is cultivating a soft uneven beard. "I thought I knew her," he says, a hint in his voice of one who has been deliberately deceived. The idea of his sister behaving without a trace of rational intention is unfathomable to him, as it was to me at first. In a single stroke her identity has changed; and by extension ours, as a family, has changed too. I detect in him the same question I keep asking: Where has she gone?

Horrified, he describes a patient he encountered while on his way to Sally's room: a round, wild-haired, gap-toothed woman devouring a mango.

"Fabulosa," I say.

"You know her?"

"I've been spending a lot of time here."

"This can't be good for Sally, identifying with these people, I mean. She's not like Fabulosa, Pops. This isn't the crowd she should be told she belongs to. Think about it, by putting her here, we're telling her she's crazy."

He drapes an arm around me. "You look like shit." Then, lowering his voice, he repeats my own dashed belief that psychedelic drugs are the cause of Sally's altered state. "I've seen people flip out after bad trips at school. It shakes them up. But they come back."

When I tell Aaron that I've already looked into this possibility, he is unconvinced. "You didn't get to the bottom of it," he says. "If she took acid, she has every reason not to come clean to you about it. She's afraid of how angry you'll be; and she wouldn't want to rat out her friends. She'll feel freer to confide in me. Watch."

And with that he goes back into her room without me, carefully closing the door.

Aaron the rescuer. I am moved by his impulse to prove that Sally doesn't really belong here.

I spot Dr. Mason coming out of the staff room.

"Has Sally been tested for substance abuse?" I ask her.

"She had a toxicology screen, yes, Mr. Greenberg. On being admitted. It's standard procedure. She was completely clean."

When Aaron emerges from Sally's room, he throws his arms around me.

"Just as I thought. She dropped acid, Pops. She was out with a bunch of friends, trying to keep up with them. Don't let on that I told you, she swore me to secrecy. She's afraid you'll never forgive her. 'Father will hate me for lying,' she says. 'Father wants to put an end to everything. He's so sad. Do you think I've made him sad?' She calls you 'Father' now, for some reason. It's a little freaky. You've got to talk to her more, Pops, try not to show how worried you are. The important thing is, she's not insane. It's just a bad trip. A very bad trip."

He embraces me again, taller, stronger than me, the body bequeathed to him by his mother's Swedish stock.

"You're crying, Pops."

"Am I?"

He looks amazed. "I never saw that before."

We go into Sally's room. "She's dead to the world," he whispers. "That's for the good. She'll probably be more herself tomorrow. Can you talk to the doctors about all the drugs they're giving her? They seem as bad for her as what landed her here. I wish they'd just give it a chance to run its course."

I break the news to him of my conversation with Dr. Mason.

"It's not possible. They must have the wrong results." He pauses, stricken. "She was so convincing. I don't see how she could have made it up." He takes me through the details of her "trip": the playground and the Sunshine Cafe, the potentially fatal certainty that she could stop moving cars—the same simple yet fantastical events that I have gone over time and again in my mind.

"Everything she told you is true," I say. "Except for the acid. She didn't take anything."

"Why would she lie to me?"

"She probably doesn't think of it as a lie. She may have thought she was keeping you safe—hard as that may be to believe. She figures we can't handle the truth. *Her* truth."

"She's right, I can't."

I can feel him gauging how implicated he is in Sally's breakdown, racing through the stages I too raced through but with a sibling's tilt. Was he too cruel to her when she was a child? "I teased her. I made fun of her weird ways. How can I be sure I wasn't the one who pushed her over?"

"You did what every brother does to his younger sister," I assure him.

HURRY DOWN SUNSHINE MICHAEL GREENBERG

We go into the dayroom, where patients in various stages of disintegration and recovery wander about.

"We can't allow her to belong to this."

"We don't look much different," I joke.

But we do look different, and with Aaron next to me the dayroom feels outlandish and raw. Fabulosa, with a purple do-rag around her head, acts as if she is in love with Aaron, mooning over him and laughing. Mitchell, a young man whose ambition to become a librarian was interrupted by schizophrenia, winks significantly at us, then apologizes for the impingement. "I didn't mean to menace you," he says. The patients ignore each other for the most part, but with a gentleness that seems connected in some way to their split-open selves. Aaron notices this too. "They live together, yet apart."

I urge him to tell me more about Youngstown, and a certain excitement creeps back into his voice. "I feel like I'm just kicking into gear, Pops. While Sally—" He stops, catching himself. "I feel relieved that it's not me in this place, and I feel guilty for feeling relieved. I wish I knew what to do for her."

"Go back upstate. Write your paper. I can't wait to read it." I promise him that we'll stay in close touch; Sally won't be on the ward forever. "They don't hold patients for very long nowadays."

In the evening I am standing in front of the supermarket on Hudson Street waiting for my brother Steve. It is time again to supply him with the eggs and frozen vegetables and canned soups and stews that he requires to survive. We have been meeting at this market since our father died two years ago, and it is with effort that I banish from my mind the image of Aaron meeting Sally in this manner thirty years from now, her maintenance one of his routine chores, the way Steve's is one of mine.

Half an hour passes and Steve still hasn't shown up. He canceled our last meeting, phoning to inform me that he wasn't feeling well, and refusing my offer to bring the food to his apartment. This was surprising. He has always been bitterly dependent on our meetings, arriving urgently with a list of new things he wants me to buy. I have come to take for granted a certain consistency from Steve, though this may be nothing more than my impatient determination not to be sucked too deeply into his world. This is who he is, I've told myself. He can't be changed. And look, his solitary life is not without its pleasures: fried eggs and tea when he wakes up at half past noon; the Woody Allen and Humphrey Bogart movies that he watches over and over again with undiminished absorption; his weekly tins of tobacco and his Barcalounger with its tilting foot rest . . .

I call him from a pay phone and a strange voice answers. I don't recollect Steve ever entertaining a visitor in his apartment.

I ask if he is there.

"Who wants to know?"

"His brother Michael."

"I heard all about you, Mister Brother."

"Are you a friend?" I ask, and immediately the word throws me: as far as I am aware, Steve has not had a "friend" since he was twelve.

"Would I be here if I was his fucking enemy?"

Possibly, I think. And in a rankled, guilty flash I see Steve as he was when we last met: with lighter burns on the tips of his fingers and his jeans stiff with grime, convinced that supermarket employees had hidden their stock of Lipton's tea for no reason other than their spiteful wish to deprive him of what he desired.

The owner of the voice hands Steve the phone, and I hear my brother's glum, belligerent "Yeah?"

"I have good news," I say. "The shelves are filled with jumbo boxes of Lipton's. I'm looking at them right now. We'll pick up an extra one so you won't be caught short. Now tell me something. Why aren't you here? I've been waiting since eight-thirty."

"Don't fuck with me, Mikey. I'm under a lot of pressure right now."

"What kind of pressure?"

"You got to get something through your skull, little brother. I don't need you anymore."

He sounds lit up on something, dry-tongued and rattled. Hearing him, I go numb with fatigue—and resentment. That this precipitous downward slide has come at the same time as Sally's crack-up seems absurdly operatic—a comic assault plotted by a perverse librettist.

"Who answered the phone, Steve?" I ask.

"That was Junior. He works at the Greeks with me."

The "Greeks" are the owners of the florist shop for which Steve occasionally delivers flowers.

"Have you been showing up for work?"

"Fuck you, little brother! Leave me alone!"

And then the slap-in-the-face sound of the receiver being slammed into its cradle at full force.

Such explosions from Steve are relatively recent. They began after our father died, prior to which Steve's excruciating social discomfort was mostly expressed with a withdrawn, apologetic stammer. It's still startling to hear him swear. He had always seemed too tentative for words like "fuck" and "cocksucker" and, for the most part, had spent his life strategically concentrated on not drawing attention to himself. With Bernie's death, however, something inside him seemed to shift. Static for decades, his "condition," as we discreetly referred to it, entered a less predictable phase. Of Bernie's five sons, Steve was the only one who did not visit him in the hospital toward the end of his life. He seemed strangely indifferent to Bernie's failing health, and I wondered if he was incapable of grief—to open the floodgates of his staunched emotional life even an inch might drown him. Bernie had been Steve's feared and dependable source of material support—and of love. He would bark at him at the slightest provocation— "You're no damn good! You can't do anything right!"—to which Steve would lower his head as if he agreed with this dim assessment of his character and was grateful to Bernie for pointing it out to him. Behind Bernie's irascibility, however, was a saving, paternal warmth. Often he would follow his disparagements with some lordly act of largesse: a luxurious gravy-soaked meal at Bernie's favorite greasy spoon or a trip to the store for a new pair of sneakers.

"Are you planning to let me starve?" Steve asked our mother, Helen, after Bernie was buried. He phoned her at all hours to remind her of his wants: garbage bags, soap, lightbulbs, sugar. What began as a test soon turned into a form of punishment. "I need chewing gum, an ice bucket, pipe cleaners, a hair clipper." And then: "I need a comforter, an answering machine, a lamp, a fan." He became reckless and enflamed, given to blasts of verbal inhumanity that made us realize how much he had held himself in check during all his years of timid recoil.

Their interactions threw Helen into an agony of panic. Seeing their mutual despair, I volunteered to take over the job of caring for him. Both Helen and Steve embraced the suggestion.

After hanging up the phone, I head uptown to Steve's apartment at Twenty-second Street and Ninth Avenue. The building is a twenty-story white brick pile that seems unsure whether it wants to look like a Holiday Inn or subsidized public housing. The sitting area in the glass lobby is inviting, but in the hallways upstairs the carpets are frayed and the walls smudged with hand prints and other less identifiable stains. At Bernie's behest, I moved Steve into the building back in 1975, with a rented truck and the help of one of our brothers. Although Steve was the second-eldest son, he had been the only one still living at home; at twenty-seven he had given no indication that he ever intended to leave. He had taken to wandering into our parents' room in the middle of the night, standing stiffly at the foot of their bed, peering at them as they slept. "Like a figure in a wax museum," said Helen. "I couldn't bear it." Bernie would order him back to his room, Steve obeying like a dismissed servant. But the next night he would be there again. "I swear to God, I was waiting for him to kill me," said Helen. Finally, Bernie gave in to her insistence that he rent Steve an apartment, something Bernie had been putting off as a financial burden "with no end in sight."

What Steve got was a one-room "studio" apartment, with light pouring through side-by-side windows on the south wall. The parquet floors had been polyurethaned to a high honey gloss, a clarion announcement of Steve's fresh start. He seemed to feel both repudiated by his forced exile from home and beguiled by the brand new pad that had been bestowed on him as—call it what it was—a payoff. It was the sheer spanking newness of the place that won Steve over. It defied resistance, like a new car. He had been kitted out with everything he would need, including the pleather Barcalounger that Bernie had presciently gone out of his way to acquire. As soon as we set it in place, Steve sat down in it like a man lowering himself into a warm bath. Every time I visited him he sat in that lounger, sucking on his pipe and drinking Lipton's tea from the pickle jar that today, twenty years later, he continues to use.

Now, I ride up to the fourth floor and knock on his door. He opens it a crack and sidles out into the hall, closing the door behind him in an obvious attempt to block my entry.

"What's the matter, Mikey? You look like you've been worked over by the Israeli army." A preemptive insult, meant to deflect attention from his own alarming appearance. I have never seen him this ravaged, yellow and rail-thin, with the exception of his chest, which juts out like a barrel whose quarter hoop is about to burst, an early symptom of emphysema. His hair is the length of a four-day beard, buzz-cut with the battery-operated clipper that after weeks of his wearying imprecations I'd bought for him. His small dry eyes dart about like he's just fled the scene of a crime and expects to be collared at any moment. On the left side of his temple is a dried brownish gash.

"Did you do your laundry?" I ask lamely.

"My laundry! Why are you so interested in my laundry? My fucking underwear! My skivvies!"

"You're filthy, Steve. Look at yourself. I gave you twenty bucks to wash your clothes."

He thrusts out his head to within inches of mine, as if daring me to sock him.

"Who are you to tell me I should wash my fucking clothes? You're nobody. Do you hear me? *Nobody*. My little cocksucking motherfucking brother, trying to be like Dad. You're not Dad. You're nothing like Dad. So fuck you! Did you hear what I said? *Fuck you!* I don't need my little brother to take care of me."

Behind me I hear a brisk metallic snap: the neighbor across the hall double-locking her door.

"It's disgusting the way you talk, Steve. The entire floor can hear you."

He is breathing loudly with a sickly wheeze, drawing on his unlit corncob pipe, furiously scratching his head, and telling me he has "a lot of problems, Mikey, more than you know, now fuck off!" He tries to duck into the apartment, but I push myself through the door after him, staggered by an onslaught of thick hot sour odors that bring tears to my eyes. Three bodies are sprawled out on woolen blankets on the floor. One, a bony woman of indeterminate age, appears to be sound asleep, as does the crumpled man beside her wearing a New York City Parks Department cap, from under which push a few sprays of white hair. On a neighboring blanket lies a large-bodied man with a lit Newport in one hand and a quart of Crazy Horse malt liquor in the other.

"I'd like you to meet my friends, Mikey. Good people. Solid people. I made some friends." And Steve proudly presents me to Junior, who, he claims, once played varsity football at Lincoln High School. "Offensive lineman, a heavy hitter, a star, Mikey. All-city."

"Yo," says Junior, offering me a swig of his Crazy Horse which I decline.

Steve seizes it, taking a loud exaggerated gulp. He is beaming: the perfect host.

"It looks like your friends are living here, Steve."

"They're visiting. Visiting! Visiting! I can guess what you're thinking, little brother, but you're dead wrong. They're not out to hurt me. I'm not their fucking *moral obligation*, their *burden*, like I am to you. I'm their friend. Their *friend*. Ever hear of voluntary emotion, little brother? I didn't think so. It makes you nervous." He laughs his coarse mirthless laugh, and continues in a stammerless rush. "I'm not saying you're mentally ill, Mikey. But you've always been so lonely, and when you're lonely you're liable to let any terrible thing climb into your head. You got to learn to trust people. They don't always stand in your way. They don't always try to keep things from you and fuck you over. Sometimes they share. Oh yes they do."

Between the belongings of Steve's "visitors" and his own accumulation of paperbacks, dirty laundry, tobacco tins, pennies, and boxes of buttons from forgotten political campaigns ("Beame's the One!"), it is almost impossible for me to venture farther into the apartment. The Barcalounger is worn down to its metal and fibrous innards. Steve has finally broken the lounger's spell, he has joined the action. He has traded his sole source of social status—this single secure room that has stood between him and the mole people, the heating grates, the park benches and midnight subway cars—for the companionship of this crowd. Stacked five feet high in the bathroom, the kitchenette, around the bed, and in just about every unused inch of the place are what appear to be the salvaged carcasses of obsolete electronic equipment: turntables, stereos, tape decks, amps, microwave ovens, answering machines . . . Some of them, however, are still in their original boxes, and I wonder if Steve's apartment is being employed to stash stolen goods.

Steve explains the clutter as "merchandise" for a "commercial enterprise" in which he is a "full and active" partner. "We haul it down to St. Marks Place. At midnight. Everybody does it. You just lay out your merchandise on the street and you're open for business. When you have inventory, Mikey, people know who you are. The cops, they look the other way after midnight."

"You should check it out," says Junior.

"You really should!" says Steve. "Stick around. It's a bazaar. We'll be heading over in a couple of hours. Garbage is money. Dad knew that, with his scrap metal yard. Scrap is garbage too. The afterlife of what has been thrown away."

He tucks a huge speaker under one arm and a monstrous amp under the other, his face growing blue from the effort, his small wrinkled muscles bulging. "I can carry this stuff all the way across town. I'm a powerhouse, Mikey."

He puts the merchandise down and stands stoop-shouldered, with his head pushed forward and his lower lip slumped out and trembling. The only light in the room is cast by Junior's cigarette and a low-wattage bulb in the bathroom, a darkness that reminds me of Steve's attraction to unilluminated rooms as a young boy. I see him as he was in those days, five years older than me, with his timid inaudible stammer. I was drawn to him then in a way that my other brothers were not—his endurance for solitude, his stillness. He seemed always to be slipping away to some unfrequented corner of our home, where, at age five or seven I would spy on him, captivated by his hunted look and his fairness: he was the only one of us with golden hair.

"I know you think I never tried to make friends. That was my disease, I brought it on myself. I know that you and Dad believed this. But look at me, Mikey. I'm trying to hack it. And you just want to take it away and fuck me. You expect me to sit alone in this fucking room, with nobody, with nothing, until I fucking die. Dad used to tell me, 'You'll never have friends. You can't be a normal person without friends.' If he was alive, he wouldn't be able to say that anymore. Would he, Mikey?"

I try to appeal to his sense of self-preservation, invoking the term "supervised living," which I know he dreads.

"If you continue like this you'll lose your independence, everything you've managed to hold on to all these years. Steve, are you listening to me?"

I wait for some indication that I have gotten through. But nothing is getting through. Junior takes another swig of his Crazy Horse, bored apparently with my impotent entreaties. I feel peculiarly distant and uninvolved. I know I should take some action, but what constitutes "action" in the case of a chronically rattled forty-eight-year-old man? I have no way to dislodge Junior or the two sleepers on the floor. I certainly can't call the police without running the risk of harming Steve, especially if some of this "merchandise" is stolen.

I manage to squeeze further into the room past a heap of teetering wire-sprouting stereo tuners, to where Junior—a large, powerful man gone mostly to fat—is enjoying his cocktail.

I pick up the gym bag that I assume contains his belongings and throw it at him, hunkering down close to him and lowering my voice to the fiercest register I can conjure. "You're not fooling me," I tell him. "I can see exactly what you and your cohorts are doing, fucking my brother over, using his place as a crash pad where you can stash your hot goods and get stoned. It's like taking advantage of a child. You hear me, Junior? I want you to clear out this instant, and drag these sorry-ass dope fiends with you. Maybe you don't know how sick my brother is. He's on medication, heavy medication, life support—drugs, alcohol, they can kill him, and if they do you'll be liable for manslaughter. I want to make sure you understand that. Manslaughter. Mandatory five to ten years."

"Steven is sick?" he asks. "You saying he's sick? I know he's sick. We're all sick. That's why we're here." He laughs. "I appreciate your concern for him. He's family, you're doing right by him, but you don't need to worry. Because Junior's watching out for him now. You got my word on that. Just ask your brother."

At Bank Street Pat is absorbed in a book of Piranesi etchings of "prisons": vaulted imaginary spaces that suggest ruined basilicas, majestically cruel with their pulleys and draw-bridges and iron posts with chains. Her notebook is open, filled with choreographic notations and phrase fragments that can be understood from inside Pat's train of thought but not mine.

She gives me the clipped obligatory "Hi" of one who doesn't wish to be interrupted.

The phone rings. It's Robin.

"There's a full moon tonight, Michael. I wish you could see it. Hanging right over the chicken coop. Like in a painting by Chagall."

"What a nice picture."

"A haunting picture. I've been trying to write down my memories. I want to collect them, to get in touch with happier times. Please tell me how our girl is doing."

As best I can, I describe Sally's recent forays into the day-room. "She's leaving her bed more than before. And Aaron's visit seemed to cheer her. All positive signs, one would think. Maybe she's getting better in ways I'm incapable of seeing."

"Better is such a relative term. She's turned herself inside out, Michael. She's cast off all restraints."

"She certainly has."

"Well, if you're going to be sarcastic." She pauses. "Look, you're on the scene with her. I can only imagine what you're going through."

"It can't be any easier for you."

"Thank you, Michael." She makes me listen to her breath for a moment, gazing, I imagine, at the Chagallian moon. "Do you remember the year Sally was born and we rented that wonderful house in Maine? Sally was a month old. She was a terrible sleeper, I was beside myself, nothing I did to put her down for the night seemed to work. The other mothers I knew told me to let her cry, she would fall asleep on her own. It was the party line. 'You have to protect yourself or there will be no end to it. You can't let the child set the agenda. You'll lose your identity. You'll resent your baby. It'll be a disaster for both of you.' They were very convincing. So I gave it a try, and after half an hour that poor baby was shaking like a wet puppy, and shrieking too, in a way I've never heard anyone shriek, not before or after. It frightened me, Michael. 'I don't know this girl,' I thought. 'I'll never know her.' This may sound crazy, but do you think this could have been what did it to Sally? My leaving her alone that night, I mean, my letting her cry."

"No. It's impossible," I say. Yet I too have difficulty bringing light to the past, let alone coaxing from it a reasonable explanation for Sally's madness. Nothing seems directly connected to it; there is no event or even series of events I can point to that might have definitively forewarned us, no obvious cause other than the most obvious one that Sally, like Steve, has always been what she has become, that it was inside her from the beginning, incubating, waiting to mature.

"But it might have been what did it," says Robin. "How can you be sure?"

"I just don't think it happens that way. Millions of babies cry without growing up to be psychotic. Look, Rob, I'm just as tempted as you are to torment myself with every little mistake we made. Aaron is too. He wondered if he had *teased* Sally into madness."

Our conversation ends.

Pat is still studying Piranesi, her hands wrapped around a steaming mug of tea. I marvel at her concentration—can she really be so thoroughly involved in her work? She seems wary of me, almost supercilious. She is so scrupulous about keeping her thoughts from me that I've given up trying to figure out what goes on inside her.

Hoping to find some relief from the heat, I carry a sleeping bag up to the roof, spread it over the welted tar, and lie down. Closing my eyes, I feel as if I've misplaced something that I mustn't lose, and jerkily sit up as if to assure myself it's still there.

At around two in the morning I come back downstairs and turn on the television. TWA flight 800, bound for Paris from JFK Airport in New York, broke apart in the air twelve minutes after taking off. "We saw a huge red orange sphere just erupt," says a private pilot who was on a pleasure flight when he saw the explosion. "It went straight down like a rock." A C-130 transport plane circles over the wreckage, dropping parachute flares to illuminate the scene for the Coast Guard search units in the water. "You think you can be hardened if you do this enough," says an Emergency Medical Service technician, "but you stay the way you are. Only more so."

On the psych ward I am lulled into the belief that this will be the routine of my life indefinitely—from Bank Street to the hospital on a continuous hypnotized track. My tense encouraging smile is a fixture in the dayroom. "Father, you are farther away than yesterday," remarks Sally.

At around three, I take a break from my visiting duties

and go out to the Recovery Room, a bar near First Avenue. It is a meeting place for operating room nurses who go there to get sloshed after long mornings at work, trading battle stories and railing against the ineptitude of surgeons. They're a promiscuous, riotous bunch, on shouting terms with death, and I enjoy listening to them from my stool at the other end of the bar. I drink two glasses of bourbon, and though my stomach is empty, the alcohol has practically no effect on me. I'm in the grip of an unshakable sobriety, compensation perhaps for the psychic drunkenness of Sally. It is as if her crack-up has made me saner than I wish to be, and I am holding on to her sober self, her other self, which she has temporarily misplaced or left behind. When she is ready I will hand it back to her, I imagine, and she will come out from under her ruinous sun and be the girl I knew again, and we will resume our pre-manic conversation. In the meantime, I am prohibited from letting go.

On the television above the bar comes news from the presidential campaign trail, candidates Bob Dole and Bill Clinton crossing the country to appear at staged events that seem, in Dole's case, to be agonizing and surreal. Dole's wry stillborn smile has a soothing effect on me that I don't fully understand. In his flawless Brooks Brothers suit, with his dyed-black 1940s-style hair, he is a man from an earlier time. In his right hand, which is maimed from a war wound, he grips a plastic pen, to keep the hand from splaying open in front of the cameras and revealing its uselessness to the world. Dole was hit by a German machine gunner in Italy in 1945, three weeks before the Nazis surrendered, during a battle that had no effect whatever on the outcome of the war. The senselessness of his wound seems connected to the futility of his presidential campaign: every day he plunges further in the polls. I picture him at the age of eighteen, returning home from the front to his small Midwestern prairie town, like the character Krebs in Hemingway's story "Soldier's Home." "People seemed to think it was rather ridiculous for Krebs to be getting back so late," after the greeting of heroes was over, Hemingway wrote. "His town had heard too many atrocity stories to be thrilled by actualities."

I dislike Dole's politics, yet watching him on the barroom television, I find myself increasingly drawn to him, with his lame arm and his noble effort to conceal it, his pinched expression of perpetually suppressed pain. The arm is like a side-kick—the ventriloquist's puppet—stealing the show, mocking the unbearable repetitions of his stump speech. "Can he close the sale with the American people?" a newscaster asks. Another wonders about his "inner anger," and his "deep sarcasm about existence."

When Dole shares the stage with Clinton, my sympathy for him sharpens. Clinton's unrelenting sunniness fills me with unease. His bright laughter, with his head thrown back, seems vaguely dangerous. Like Samuel Coates, the superintendent of America's first lunatic asylum, I have come to distrust "the uncertainty of all human exaltation."

The operating room nurses at the bar are talking loudly, fresh from a kidney transplant. "Who's your daddy?" one of them asks me with a slightly cockeyed leer. She means: Who is the monkey on my back, the person I can't throw off? Who has my number?

I search her face for signs of aberrance, the bent glow I

have grown accustomed to seeing on the ward. After a brief exchange, she accuses me, with a hint of contempt, of being "a civilian," and turns back to her friends.

On the screen above the bar, Bob Dole is now at a campaign rally, pursued by hired hecklers dressed in enormous foam-rubber cigarette costumes. "Tobacco is no worse for you than milk!" they chant, repeating one of the gaffes that have helped to derail his campaign. He holds his right arm tight to his body, bent at the elbow, just enough to give the illusion that it isn't maimed. To me, it is the sum total of who he is, the source of what I have construed to be his brave comfortless control. He seems bitterly amused by the cigarette protest, as if he doesn't care about the election anymore. He knows it is lost. "I've taken a vow of silence," he says. "My handlers have muzzled me. They claim that every time I open my mouth I lose more votes for the Republican party."

I return to the hospital to resume the wait for Sally's monstrous ebullience to pass.

The following day my mother is at the ward, standing in the sweltering hall outside Sally's room with Pat and me.

"Michael, why did you keep this from me?" she asks, squeezing my hand with punitive sympathy. "If Pat hadn't phoned this morning I'd still be in the dark. This has to be some kind of mistake. That gorgeous girl. Tell me it's a mistake."

"I felt Helen should know," explains Pat. "We've kept it to ourselves for too long."

"You certainly have. Michael, I've never seen you like this.

Your eyes look like Peter Lorre's in that Fritz Lang movie, what was it called?"

"M," I say, grateful to have her with us, with her worrying ways thinly disguised as humor—her comedy of pain.

"Yes!"

"Steve had a similar reaction to my appearance."

"He's a fine one to talk."

She is perfectly turned out in a pair of white-and-caramel heels and a honey-colored linen suit with a small golden frog pinned to the lapel. Her blonded hair is freshly coiffed, her neck concealed under a weightless, diaphanous scarf with the names of Riviera resort towns floating on it: an American Catherine Deneuve.

When we enter her room, Sally effusively greets her "nanny," spreading her arms to present her glorious self for inspection, looking for all the world like a cheerful teenage girl.

"I know why you're here."

"Of course you do. I'm here to see you, sweetheart." And with a reproachful glance at me, Helen says: "She looks wonderful, Michael."

"I *am* wonderful, aren't I. I was counting on you to see it, Nanny. Not like him." Sally narrows her eyes at me: "Father, you're the only one who is still in the dark." And rising from her bed, she walks imperiously out into the hall.

As we follow her, past the nurse's station and the bustling glass-walled staff room, Helen grips my arm.

"She's just a little overwrought. It's probably hormonal. Hyperthyroid, you know what I mean. *Hayva buttel*, your grandmother Yetta would have called it in Yiddish. Taking a breather." And she resurrects the case of a childhood neighbor whose racing pituitary gland briefly caused her father to mistake her for a lunatic. "Who *doesn't* lose it for a while at Sally's age? Only the most frighteningly boring girls. You should have seen yourself at fifteen, Michael, you almost sent us all to the asylum."

"But she's suffering," I say, and then immediately wonder if this is true or if it is *our* plight to suffer, while Sally barrels ahead without feeling, like a runaway train.

Helen catches up to Sally as she enters the dayroom. "Tell your father you're not suffering."

"The truth comes disguised as suffering. My father has been destroyed by fear."

"Your father is worried about you, sweetheart. It's only natural."

"Hmmm. You're trying to protect him. That's to be expected. He's your precious son, isn't he, Nanny? Or are you trying to trick me, and you are afraid too?"

Helen looks like she's been slapped in the face. She takes my hand, digging her nails into my flesh.

"She'll get over it, Michael. As God is my witness, this will pass. In ten, fifteen years, when she's married and working at a job that she loves, you'll look back on this as a blip on the screen."

A handsome man of about sixty in a rumpled suit approaches us—a man of culture by all appearances, with a rising Beethovenian forehead and flowing, thick, steel-gray hair.

"Are you visiting someone?" Helen politely asks.

"You mean, 'Do you live here?' Isn't that what you're asking? 'Is this where you belong?'"

"Oh!" And with a sideways giggle, fiddling with her scarf, she says to Pat and me, "I didn't realize he was one of the meshugah. He looks so . . . *intelligent*. I guess you can never be sure."

Despite our protests—that she needn't upset the rhythm of her life so thoroughly, much less subject herself to the discomforts of the ward—Helen shows up in Sally's room every day at noon. She stays for at least four hours, brushing me off when I, knowing her widow's calendar to be crammed with lunch dates and bridge games, suggest that at least she make her visits shorter. Her bright careful veneer calms us. Every day she arrives in a fresh outfit, stretching her wardrobe to the limit, not a hair out of place or a hint of summer wilt about her. She enters the ward as if she's stepping onto a stage, but it seems less a display of vanity than a tribute to order, to effort, to the way we must will things to be in times of disaster. The harder the blow, the more polish is required, she seems to be saying, as if her suits and pleated skirts amount to an ethical rejection of chaos. Some of the female staffers seem flattered by the care she takes in her appearance, feeling it is for them as well. "You are one royal lady," Cynthia Phillips tells her. And even Rufus treats her to a respectful nod of his head when he unlocks the door.

Sometimes I doubt whether Sally even notices our presence; at other times she tantalizes us with glimmers of coherence that dim as suddenly as they arise. False calls. On certain afternoons she is awake for no more than an hour, and the three of us—Pat, Helen, and I—fall into the almost pleasurable rhythm of the ward, its detained unchanging crawl. When I question why we're sitting here without her, I tell myself: If we weren't waiting for her to come back to us, she would lose the sense that there was a point of return.

Helen, for her part, seems determined to embrace our distress as her own. It occurs to me that this is precisely what she is here for, that she has turned herself over to this place—to us—as a way of reexperiencing what she went through with Steve. She is here as Sally's grandmother, of course, as a supporting presence in a time of familial crisis, but she is also making amends with herself, I think, as if, by passing all these hours with us, a harsh frozen fact from her past can be softened or thawed.

"What's a five-letter word for a sacred Buddhist text that begins with the letter s?" Helen asks, folding the day's crossword puzzle in her lap like a freshly ironed napkin.

"Sutra," says Pat, earning a delighted grin from Helen.

We haven't spent such concentrated amounts of time in each other's company since I was a boy. As adults, our relationship has been uneasy—the lasting effect of a rupture that occurred between us when I was eleven or twelve, and that we have never managed fully to repair. And yet, shielded by Pat's presence, and bolstered by the feeling of solidarity that Sally's crack-up has inspired, we are able, provisionally at least, to overcome our awkwardness with each other. The three of us make interminable small talk, and take aimless arm-in-arm strolls up and down the halls. Helen recounts the plots of movies she has recently seen, Pat tells stories about her Irish grandmother who ran a numbers racket and rarely let her rosary out of her hands, and the two of them argue amicably about the relative merits of New York City Ballet's principal dancers. Slowly, the air of solemnity lifts from our afternoons. The ward begins to feel more like a nursery than a prison, a refuge where one is removed from pressure, expectation, and, with the help of meds and electroshock, from memory as well. We plan luncheon picnics in the dayroom, where we hang out amid the hubbub of the patients and their families. "The piazza," Helen calls it.

When she's feeling up to it, Sally joins us. "I tried calling Mom," she says. "I dialed 1-802. *One ate oh too*," she says, miming the words. "Do you see why I couldn't go on?"

One afternoon Pat leaves the ward early, to go to a rehearsal of her dance company, and Helen and I find ourselves alone. Immediately our customary awkwardness returns. With Sally knocked out and nothing to distract us, our conversation deteriorates into an excruciating series of false starts. This tense embarrassed shyness can be traced back to the fall of 1964, when I destroyed the close bond between Helen and me that was the envy of my older brothers, who retaliated with covert acts of revenge that left me terror-struck and in constant miserable expectation of a fresh attack. My status as Helen's favorite even incited a certain grumpiness in my father. I had become a pariah, a mama's boy. Only Steve left me alone, as he left everyone alone; yet without saying a word he seemed to reproach me more severely than the others for the special attentions I enjoyed. He needed them more. I had her all for myself, "staying home" on the basis of some "flu" or invented fever (while Bernie was at his scrap metal yard and my brothers at their desks in school) so Helen could take me to matinee movies and then to a soda fountain on Flatbush Avenue for grilled cheese sandwiches and cantaloupe halves. I don't remember the details of my rejection of her, only the violent feeling, and the verbal cruelty I unleashed upon her without warning or the slightest regard for the blow that I was forcing her to absorb. I ordered her to steer clear of me. I tore her apart with a barrage of furious riffs that poured out of my eleven-year-old mouth in a sudden shocking eloquence of meanness—an eloquence that I was just discovering in myself and that Helen was completely unprepared for. Things were said that were hardhearted and final. What I most remember was the demonic driven feeling, and then our retreat from each other for good. For a long time I've wanted to apologize for my behavior that year, but I'm not sure how or even if it would be sincere. How does the man apologize for the boy?

At the close of visiting hours, Helen suggests that we go out to dinner. We enter the first restaurant we pass, a bar with a small dining room in the back where a few vacant tables are arranged under a murky green-tinted skylight that makes us feel as if we are sitting underwater. I order a bourbon, and Helen, who usually doesn't drink, asks for a gin and tonic. Around her neck hangs a small gold medallion engraved with the names of her five sons—a gift from our father—which she fidgets with nervously, raising her eyes to me as if she's about to speak and then turning away without muttering more than a couple of stilted words.

Our drinks arrive, two brimming cocktail glasses still warm from their rinsing at the bar sink, the ice cubes thinning fast.

"How's Steve?" she asks.

I fill her in on the latest. "I don't know what to do about him right now."

"What *can* be done at this point? He's a grown man. Your father and I wore ourselves out trying. You've been wonderful with him, Michael. If I haven't thanked you properly it's not because I'm not grateful."

"I know."

I have the powerful sense that she has thought through what she wants to say to me, and I am anxiously searching for a way to help her along, when her hands tighten around her drink and in a rising voice she says: "Sally is nothing like Steve. As God is my witness. I saw that boy grow up. I saw everything. And I swear to you, Sally is nothing like him."

She waves a hand at her finely spun hair, as if to say, *No need to utter another word about this.* But then, after sipping her drink through a red cocktail straw, and removing the straw and twisting it around her finger, she goes on.

"If what I say ends up sounding like a complaint, then I'm saying it wrong." And she launches into a complicated family history that seems to come out of nowhere at first, but that I soon realize is inextricably connected to Steve and Sally and me. I've heard some of these stories of course, they're part of our family lore, but never told to me like this, from Helen, and so startlingly meant for my ears alone.

She begins with the sudden, devastating blow of her father's death when she was thirteen ("How I wish you could have met him, Michael. He would have changed your life, I'm sure of it") and her marriage nine years later to Bernie, who had come charging onto the scene, and into her affections, as an irresistible force.

"My father was a physician, a literary man, a man of science. You'll understand me when I tell you that if he hadn't died I probably would never have met Bernie. We traveled in different circles. Bernie was—how shall I put it . . ."

"Primitive," I offer.

"That's your word, Michael. You thought we were all vulgar. You had a false notion of sophistication. Your father wasn't primitive, he was volatile, impatient—you of all people should know the difference."

And yet in the next breath she grows nostalgic for the cosmopolitanism and intellectual stimulation that were abruptly withdrawn from her when her father died.

"It doesn't make me swell with pride to admit that during my first years with Bernie I felt I had made a grave mistake. We were miserable."

Her in-laws, Yetta and Louie, were illiterate, immigrants from the shtetl world of Eastern Europe, Louie a welder and ironmonger who had been fending for himself since he landed alone in New York at the age of fifteen. "Sally's age, if you can imagine it."

Newlyweds during the housing shortage of the midforties when masses of GIs were returning home from the Second World War, Helen and Bernie had no choice but to move in with them. "We weren't millionaires. There was no place else to live."

But Helen's misery wasn't the result of any residual snob-bism she may have felt or the fact that Yetta was a ferocious *balabusta* who, with Helen's agitated assistance, did nothing but chop and boil and roast and polish and scrub and mop—no, what made her life unbearable in her in-laws' apartment in Brighton Beach Brooklyn was the continuous war between Bernie and his father.

The war was for the scrap metal business that Louie had squandered his health building from scratch. "It wasn't US Steel," says Helen, "but it was Louie's, it was a temple to him, and it was just coming into its own when Bernie came aboard." By the time Louie was fifty he couldn't walk to the corner without stopping to catch his breath with his hands on his knees. He had ruined his lungs as a young man welding trash cans in a windowless basement on Grand Street. And he could see it was all going to be Bernie's, the easy money, the American boon, Bernie didn't have to give up a damn thing for it, and Louie was going to make him pay, he wasn't going to let him have it for nothing.

"He wouldn't forgive your father for taking what was sim-ply *there for him to take*. So you see, Michael, when I tell you it was war, I mean it in the most literal sense. He loved Bernie as a son and hated him as a rival, hated him, I sometimes thought, the way an immigrant hates a privileged native."

They tore each other to pieces at that scrap metal yard, and when they returned home they'd pick up where they left off. "Bernie would be just seething with emotion, battered and charged up, but depressed too, if you can imagine this combination." Once, he came home with blood dribbling out of the corner of his mouth where Louie had slugged him. "It was a nightmare for both of them, and it was a nightmare for Yetta and me too. I wanted to comfort Bernie, to make it easier for him, to soothe him, I wanted to bring him closer to me, but it was impossible, we were lost to each other, your father and I, and as a matter of fact, we were lost in ourselves."

She falls silent for a moment.

"Am I talking too much? I just want to give you a picture of how it was, Michael, the atmosphere of those years, the unhappiness. I was twenty-two."

It was into this atmosphere that my eldest brother Jay was born, giving Helen a reason to feel alive again.

"I can't tell you how much I adored that baby. He saved my life, there's no other way to put it. He *was* my life." And after describing her glorious days with Jay in that embattled home, she says flatly: "And then I became pregnant with Steve."

She felt something was wrong the minute she started carrying him. "It was like this crushed weight in me, Michael. Does that sound crazy? I was sick with the idea of having another child under those circumstances, I wanted to enjoy the one I had. Obviously something was wrong with me, not Steve. I mean, what could be at the heart of such dislike for an unborn child but contempt for myself?"

Her eyes are bright and determined, with the moist intensity I remember in them as a boy.

"If you feel like having another drink, I might decide to join you," she says.

I order another round. Our notion of having dinner has

been forgotten. I am speechless and thankful and oddly ashamed.

"I just had no love for him," she continues. "Isn't that re-markable? All I felt was resentment—resentment for this tiny *thing* that was going to invade my paradise."

She prayed that her feelings would change when he was born, that with the flesh-and-blood reality of her baby some-thing would shift inside her and nature would come to her aid. But the actuality of Steve only made matters worse.

"The fact is, he was an exceptionally beautiful child. Large-eyed, handsome, God help us, you wouldn't know it to look at him now. Total strangers would stop us on the street, other mothers, Michael, pushing their own babies, they'd stop and tell me how beautiful Steve was, 'Like a painting,' they'd say, 'a perfect angel.' And harsh judges those mothers were, every one of them an expert. Believe me, child rearing in Brooklyn was a highly competitive business."

What they didn't know was how unresponsive Steve was. "Sometimes he just went limp. I swear to you, he seemed as good as dead, except for his eyes looking up at me, intent and wide. He just lay there—not gloomy or depressed or unhappy or even crying out to me—just blankly watching me play with his older brother."

And I think: for Steve, watching them must have been like looking in at some paradisiacal garden through a crack in the wall.

"I've gone over it in my head a thousand times, and I be-lieve that Steve went limp in that way because he thought it would please me. I'm under no illusions, it was also a survival tactic, I've no doubt about it. He knew what it did to me when he made a fuss. It angered me, it distracted me from his older brother. And *he knew* it. His invisibility was a way of accommodating me. He was tuned in. He knew how I felt. Though I didn't realize this at the time."

And she tells me of leaving him out in the cold, in his carriage. "Two, three hours. I'd completely forget about him. Then I'd remember! My God! And there he would be, right in front of our building, his lips blue, his mittened fingers like ice. And he still didn't make a peep."

When Steve did cry it was a sick frightened dry cackle that was almost like being scratched. "It should have broke my heart. But what I felt was this pure rage at him for doing this to me, for turning me into this unloving monster. It got to the point where his very existence was an indictment of mine."

She drinks the melted ice that is what is left of her second gin and tonic and sets the glass down carefully, as if to make sure not to disrupt some imaginary arrangement.

"You couldn't help yourself," I say. "It wasn't intentional. It was an impossible situation. For both of you. What you had may well have been a classic case of postpartum depression."

"That's sweet of you to say, Michael. But I'm not looking to get off the hook."

Things didn't stay bad forever. The spell broke when Helen and Bernie moved into their own home in Rockaway, a narrow spit of coastland across a drawbridge from Brooklyn. It was a middle-class neighborhood, with other young families. "We made new friends, lifelong friends." Louie grew too sick to work and the scrap metal business passed on to Bernie. "That feeling of being cornered, of being walled in, lifted, thank goodness. Larry was born, and then you, and Danny. I loved my boys. And I loved your father. Even in the darkest days, it never occurred to me to leave him."

She rests her hand on my arm.

"You see, Michael, Sally is nothing like Steve. Whatever is happening to her, it isn't inherited from your brother. So please, please strike that from your list of worries. Steve is the way he is because of me."

The next day Helen skips her visit, and the day after that she comes only for an hour. "My dog has been missing me," she explains. Her confession has left us unsure of where to pick up again, even as a new ease develops between us, an unexpected gift of Sally's illness, I think.

I try to bring up the rupture that took place between us when I was a boy—an attempt to make amends. Helen pretends not to know what I'm talking about. Then, switching gears, she says: "Don't you think I understood your behavior, Michael? 'There's no winning,' I said to myself. 'This is what he has to do to believe he can be a man.' The truth is, I indulged myself with you, just like I did with your brother Jay. It's a weakness of mine. But you know, you didn't have to tear things apart so completely."

Her tone suggests that she'd just as soon forget it; it's old news.

Sensing that she is ready to return to her life as it was before, I promise to phone regularly with reports of Sally's progress.

"If something important happens, I can be there in twenty minutes," Helen says.

Although I have noticed little change in Sally, I am informed by Dr. Mason that "the most acute phase" of her mania has passed. The nurses look in on her less often and in general seem to be less worried about her taking a turn for the worse—the psychiatric equivalent of being removed from intensive care. I wonder if she is improving in increments too small for me to measure, like a caterpillar climbing a giant pole. The essence of Sally's illness, I suspect, is as unknown to Dr. Mason as it is to me. Sally's "essence," however, is not Dr. Mason's concern, the practical steps of her recovery are, and I do my best to keep up with them as we go along.

Sally sleeps less and spends more time in the dayroom, convinced that she is a great social success there. "Have you noticed how people want to be around me?" she asks. "I feel that I'm helping them. That's why Dr. Mason won't send me home. I bring hope to them, especially to the depressives. I'm their shining star."

She certainly acts like one, holding court in her gleaming pajamas. Her audience includes Mitchell, who appears to be slightly in love with her, and Fabulosa, who is covered in crumbs from tearing open packets of soup crackers with her teeth. The man with the Beethovenian forehead whom Helen mistook for a visitor eyes Sally with amusement. He is obviously in his own manic orbit, a daunting figure, electrified and bored, wearing L.L. Bean moccasins and a midnight blue pajama suit with white piping down the middle that looks as if it belonged to Cary Grant.

"Your daughter is touched by the gods," he says to me.

"The Greeks called madness 'the sacred disease,' so you can rest assured she is in good company."

He exudes a crackling fanatical aliveness that makes my heart race. It reminds me of Sally's emanations, but more mature and formed. Indeed, the similarities between them astonish me—their clenched grin, their narrow movie-villain stares. He is bear-like and imposing, and separated from Sally in age by at least forty years.

Seeing that I am drawn to him, Sally exhorts me to pay even closer heed. "He never lost touch with his genius. This is the way you could be too." But he and Sally avoid actual contact with each other, as if repelled by their competing intensities.

A young man enters the room and introduces himself to me as Dexter. "I see you've been talking with my father. I hope he didn't force himself on you. He's used to speaking to a captive audience. He's a classics professor, if he hasn't already told you as much." He names the university where his father is employed. "He'll only be here for a couple of days."

Noticing that his father is trembling slightly, Dexter leads him to a quiet corner of the dayroom. The professor, in an agony of restiveness, tightens and untightens his fists and runs both hands through his hair. He appears to be racing at full tilt. Dexter talks to him in a low voice, settling him down, I think, whispering what I imagine to be a series of private calming phrases.

Later, I run into Dexter in the hall. I find myself looking to him for news of my own future. He is a cognoscente of madness, I think, he grew up with it, to him, perhaps, it's a natural element of existence. When I tell him the story of

Sally's crack-up, he nods knowingly. He's lived it a dozen times. His father and Sally have been struck by the same lightning. "I saw your daughter at full throttle the other day. They both know how to dish it out. But when he's himself," he says of his father, "there's no gentler more considerate person in the world."

I feel a rush of hope. The professor is in a cycle, the wheel turns, he comes back to where he started. If they are really alike, then Sally will come back too, at least for a while.

Later in the afternoon, I catch sight of the professor in his room, looking blander and older. Dexter is reading to him in the same calming voice he employed in the dayroom. The professor's eyes are closed, and I have the impression that he is listening to the sound of the words, not their meaning.

A couple of days later, the professor is standing by the nurses' station wearing a silvery gray suit, newly pressed. His brogues have been freshly polished. His shirt is buttoned to the top of his neck. He is being discharged.

"I just needed to get back on track," he says in a soft voice, as if he will be reprimanded if he's overheard. "A periodic adjustment. It's why I'm here—for that mallet blow to the brain."

Dexter, for his part, is stern with his father. Look what you've put us through again, he seems to be saying. I feel as if I am witnessing a ritual that they've repeated hundreds of times.

The professor sits on a bench by the ward's entrance, like a schoolboy waiting for class to begin, while Dexter collects his prescriptions from Nurse Phillips. He invites me to sit beside him. "Dexter wants my money. He won't be satisfied until he has me declared permanently *beside myself*. My retirement account, the apartment. Don't fool yourself. He has calculated to the penny how much he stands to gain."

Sally comes out of her room. "You're going home! Good for you!"

Dexter and I shake hands. He is bracing himself for the long pull back to recovery. He knows the drill: his father smashed to pieces after the sparkle of his mania has dimmed. "He hates the halting dullness that comes over him after an attack. He feels ashamed." Dexter will remind him of what he's made of his life: the students he's inspired, the books he's written, the great original intelligence that is his to call on whenever he feels the spirit. "The real joy he's given to people. Including me. *Especially* me."

Neither of us suggests that we stay in touch. An acquaintance struck up on the psych ward doesn't leave it.

"Good luck, Sally," he says.

With one hand Dexter holds his father's night bag, the other he rests on his shoulder, guiding him through the door which Rufus has unlocked.

Sally is moved to a room that she will share with two other patients, at the end of a long hall, far from the command posts of the staff room and the nurse's station. "A graduation," Dr. Mason tells me with a strained smile. "A sign of her improving state of mind."

The new room is pleasant and large, renovated in the manner of a student dorm. Sally inhabits it as a starlet would her hotel suite, her voice powerful and distinct, but oddly unreal, like a recording of herself she is playing back to me. One of her roommates is a teenage girl from Harlem who lies inertly on her bed with the covers piled over her in a chaotic mound. Her mother has decorated the wall above her bed with yellow smiley faces and get well cards and happy crayon drawings that, the mother told me, the girl made as a child.

Her inertia tugs at me like a magnet. Blues like this lives out of sight of the world, I think. It seems more a solid organic mass than a mood that can blow away or be lifted. It lies there and says, *Go ahead, try to budge me.*

I drop my voice so as not to disturb her, then realize that I am the only one bothering to make such an adjustment. No one else in the room pays her any mind. Blues like this doesn't have ears. It can't be disturbed. It has nothing to do with sadness or even grief—which at least are imaginable emotions.

Sally has settled cheerfully into her new digs. She seems to regard the change as a coronation. "I'm a positive example," she says, repeating words she has picked up during group therapy sessions on the ward. "I'm the kind of person they want around their clients." She insists on her health, outlining her plans to join the hospital staff as a therapist, and also to become a nursery school teacher—one job to help adults refind themselves, the other to teach children to hold on to their perfect souls. "I'm going to enter a beauty pageant," she says. "I'm going to become a dancer, like you, Pat." My heart rises when she allows Pat to hold her for a few seconds, Pat reassuring her much as Dexter reassured his father.

She strikes up an excited friendship with her second roommate, a garrulous woman from the suburbs of Long Island with two small children at home. The woman defies me to believe that just three months ago anorexia had brought her so close to death she was being fed through a tube. She makes her bed without a single crease, like the bunk of a marine, and she is surrounded by photographs of her rotund Italian-American clan. She offers us tiny plastic spoonfuls of tiramisu like someone giving away samples in a store. "A gift from my sister," she says. "Isn't it sublime?"

On the day of her release her husband comes to take her home. Her cheerfulness seems to worry him, her repeated declarations that her life has been set straight, that what ailed her is over now, "a chapter from my past." Her husband and I exchange thin apprehensive smiles, while Sally helps her pack, the two of them chattering like conspirators. He is a lineman for the Long Island Lighting Company and is exhausted from working long hours in the summer heat wave.

"You'll be with your family!" says Sally.

The depressed girl lies in her bed in a granite silence, unignorable yet ignored.

The following afternoon we are informed that in a few days Sally too will be discharged. A social worker, Julian, is assigned to help "facilitate a smooth transition" from the psych ward to the "less supervised environment" of Bank Street. He informs me that prior to Sally's discharge there will be a meeting with him and Dr. Mason. "It would be best if Sally's mother could be there. And her brother." The purpose of the meeting, he explains, is to promote an atmosphere of understanding of Sally's "changed circumstance," her "special needs."

"I've located an outpatient program that may be just the ticket for Sally after she's released," he says. "I'll have more information at our meeting." He has the halting speech of one who has overcome a childhood stammer. Knowing that I am a writer, he bashfully tells me that he too is an artist—a cellist—social work is his backup profession, the freelance life was too stressful, the self-abnegation it required, the raw tests of endurance and nerves. "I guess I caved," he says.

I take the sympathy that flows between us as a good omen and permit myself to worry aloud about what lies in store for Sally, fishing for tidbits of information that Julian may have overhead among the staff.

"What is it you want for her?" he asks.

The directness of the question jars me, and I hear myself wishing for the return of what has been demolished in her, if it ever really existed. "A center, I guess is what one normally calls it, where she can check on herself, even if she doesn't pay it any heed." I wonder if such a basic and ineffable thing can be built, like a prosthetic, or learned through a series of exercises the way one learns algebra or a second language. "If only I could give this to her," I say.

I reach Robin at her bakery in Vermont. "I'm in the middle of making a wedding cake. It's like building someone's dream house. I can't get the icing right. I'm on my fourth batch, ready to fall off my feet."

She sounds exhilarated. Her wedding cakes are famous in Vermont. She is a gifted baker, just as she is gifted at most things she turns her hand to.

"How is she, Michael? It's impossible to get through to her. I dial the number Nurse Phillips gave me and it just rings and rings."

"They're discharging her the day after tomorrow," I say. It hits me how much I have been dreading this: Sally under our sole care. I tell Robin about the family meeting that is to take place prior to Sally's release. "They'd like us all to be there."

"I'll finish the cake tonight and drive down. George will come with me. I want him to be part of this too. To show our togetherness, Michael. To Sally, but also to each other."

"Of course."

I hear the whir of her electric mixer. It would be nice to be able to bake, I think, "building" a cake as Robin calls it, erecting this enormous symbolic dessert that will be photographed and enshrined in a leather-bound album, and that will be eaten with music and champagne and applause.

"We didn't have a cake at our wedding," I remark.

"We weren't thinking about cakes."

True enough. We were preparing for Aaron, who would be born in less than a month. Robin's wedding gown was a maternity dress. Our wedding was for him. Our part in it was an afterthought. *We* were an afterthought, even to ourselves.

In the morning I wake Aaron in his student house in Schenectady.

"I'll be there, Pops. I'm glad she's getting out of that place. She doesn't belong with those people. The sooner she's home, the better."

We meet up with Robin and George at a coffee shop near the hospital, George in shorts, sandals, a green chamois shirt, the two of them cleaved together in their window booth, a display case of marital harmony.

"Sally's way out there," says George. "But hey, so are a lot of great people." He's a minister's son with an enduring interest in mysticism, football, and ganja. The sticker on the tailgate of his Ford pickup says: A Good Patriot Must Defend His Country Against Its Government. It was startling to note, the first time I saw them together, how much more suited than I George was to being Robin's husband. She seemed more sure of herself with him, less surrendering and dreamy. It became clearer than ever to me that I had thwarted her in some way, exhorting her to stick to painting, though the pressure to be an artist was obviously disturbing to her. I couldn't accept the fact that Robin was so nonchalant about her natural talents, while I was struggling to figure out whether I possessed any at all.

Out on the street several men with pneumatic drills are tearing up the pavement—a painful racket that during her previous visit would have made Robin cower. In the company of George, however, she appears to be oblivious to the noise and immune to the cement dust that comes swirling at us as we leave the coffee shop and head to the ward. George clearly adores her, clasping her hand, deferring to her intelligence, admiring her in a way that I, for all my keenness for Robin, never did.

Pat, as always with those with whom she feels instinctively at odds, is impenetrably friendly. "You must be exhausted after your trip," she says. "I can imagine how difficult it was for you to get away." Her pleasantries don't ask for a reply. It's as if she's watching us through a fencer's mask.

We ride up to the ward, where Aaron is already sitting on the edge of Sally's bed, his hands planted firmly on her shoulders, delivering what appears to be a coach's pep talk. "You can get past this. You're a strong girl. The strongest. The best," he says, his eyes boring into her with an earnestness that breaks my heart. If only such exhortations could sway her. Turning to us, he says, "I was just telling Sally that when she gets home everything will fall into place. She'll have her independence again. We'll get your room ready, Sally. We'll make it special. You'll forget you were ever in this place."

"A new day," says George.

"Amen," says Robin.

Hugs all around, as Sally looks on, restless and glazed.

Her roommate lies under our radar, bundled in her mummy sheets exactly as she was the last time I was here. I notice the eyes of the others drift over to her, taking in the weight of her presence.

Julian pokes his head in. It's time for our meeting. He leads us through the hall and into a small locked conference room or lounge.

On the table is a copy of the *New York Times*.

A pipe bomb spiked with nails and screws shattered the Summer Olympic Games today in Atlanta, transforming an international event of sport and fellowship into a symbol of the dark side of modern life.

The six of us sit down like people assembled in a court-room waiting for the judge to emerge from her chambers and take her place on the bench.

Sally supplies the soundtrack, her left leg in a continuous shudder, her foot tapping the floor at lightning speed.

"Do you have children?" she asks Julian.

"As a matter of fact, I do, Sally. I have a daughter. She's almost two."

"The age of genius."

Dr. Mason comes through the door, greeting us as a single entity with a sweeping nod. "Good. You're all here. How do you feel?" she asks Sally.

"Like I'm packed in foam rubber."

"That's not surprising. You're still getting used to the medication." To us she says: "I like Sally's answer. It shows she's thinking outside of herself. She's shifting away from the literal-mindedness of psychosis where a person is not *like* God, he *is* God. Mind you, I'm not saying Sally ever thought she was God. I'm just giving the most obvious example. Do you have any thoughts about what I just said, Sally?"

"Have you decided whether I'm crazy?" she asks.

"'Crazy' is a word we prefer not to use," says Mason.

Sally's foot tapping continues, like the ticking of a rapidly turning wheel.

"This will pass when the haloperidol is adjusted," says Mason.

"When will that be?" I ask.

"That's a matter for Sally's outside doctor to deal with."

I worry aloud about the extent to which the medication

will change Sally over time. "It seems to be killing more than her psychosis."

"Well, yes, Mr. Greenberg, the medication *is* changing her. That's what it's supposed to do. There will be side effects, of course—sluggishness, some blobbing perhaps."

Beneath her supremely authoritative surface, I sense the resignation that settles on many clinical psychiatrists after a while, like a dull professional coating: the tacit, almost visible shrug that says, *This is all I can do for you*, which is the psychiatrist's cross to bear. It's easy to imagine how dispiriting it must be to administer a series of unrewarding treatments that have not progressed much since Lady Macbeth's doctor observed: "This disease is beyond my practice . . . More needs she the divine than the physician."

Aaron wants to know if the average person on the street will be able to tell that Sally is on medication.

"She won't be doing the Thorazine shuffle, if that's what you mean. But will she be the most normal-looking person on the A train? Probably not."

"How about on the 1 train?" asks Pat.

We laugh, Sally the loudest.

"At fifteen one's personality has not yet crystallized," says Mason. "Adolescents go through phases that feel . . . transformative. There are so many possibilities, so many roads not taken that may still present themselves to Sally. We don't yet know her baseline, so I can't tell how close to it she is now."

Sally's baseline: one's median behavior on the mood chart. (Who created this chart? And how can its accuracy be gauged?) The word has a strange power. *If a runner strays from the baseline he is automatically ruled out.* Is the return of Sally's baseline what I've been waiting for all these weeks? Or is Mason referring to a new normal that I haven't encountered yet, but will recognize when it makes itself known?

I look at Sally sitting across the table between Robin and Aaron, depressed or elated or in a mixed state that includes all moods at once. How would I know? She has been wrenched from the severest form of psychosis—exorcism by drugs, just enough for her to go home. But what else has been achieved?

"When she gets home don't put pressure on her," advises Mason. "Give her time." And turning to Julian, she says: "Do you remember the girl whose parents said, 'When you come home you can do this and this,' and they listed a whole calendar of activities they had set up for her, and she said, 'Yeah, all the things that put me here in the first place'? That was just perfect."

I feel as if she's just punched me in the face. With a look, I appeal to Julian who strikes a neutral, slightly embarrassed pose, not wishing to endorse Mason's comment, but wary of antagonizing her. Until now it has been a matter of tacit medical agreement that Sally's illness is purely a case of neurotransmitters that have gone haywire. However, Mason, in an unguarded aside that seems to represent her true belief, has blamed *us* for Sally's condition. The humiliating assumption is that when we take Sally home she will be returning, in the parlance of mental hygiene workers, to "a situation that is not working." As the architects of this "situation," we are promoters of psychosis. We are guilty on both counts, it seems, nature *and* nurture.

By now, my hopelessness about a medical solution is complete.

Finally, Mason delivers Sally's diagnosis. Ostensibly, this is the purpose of our meeting, but she treats it as if it is an item on an uncompleted form that must be filled in and filed. She pronounces Sally "bipolar 1," not because she places great store in this diagnosis, I think, but because Sally has to have a label, an identity card to carry her through the mental health system, and bipolar 1 will do.

In fact, it is the diagnosis I have been hoping for, because its social weight is lighter than the other diagnosis, the doomed diagnosis, schizophrenia. Manic depression (as bipolar 1 used to be called) is the affliction of Byron, Robert Schumann, Virginia Woolf—the disease of exuberance, of volatility and magnetism and invention. If only I believed this.

"I would call Sally's case classic," Mason says, "except for the fact that she is a tad young to be presenting in such an . . . adult fashion. The initial manic episode doesn't usually occur until the patient is in her twenties. The prognosis for adolescent onset can be less optimistic, but there are no rules . . ."

Her tone of voice suggests that she has already left the room, which she promptly gets up to do, the legs of her chair scraping against the floor as she rises. "You're going to be fine. Things will work out. Trust your doctor. You just need to follow the program."

There is a momentary vacuum after Mason leaves.

"Quite a piece of work," says George.

Robin sighs, as if to indicate a collective release of tension.

Encouraging and nervous, Julian says: "I've received a green light from the outpatient program, so when you leave us, Sally, you won't be stepping into a void."

He announces that we must draw up a "Wellness Contract," a set of guidelines to follow when Sally returns home. "It's a contract between Sally and you, her caregivers," he explains, removing a yellow legal pad from his briefcase and setting it on the table. "You'll find it helpful to have these things spelled out in black and white. It'll give Sally something to work toward, a feeling of progress. A goal."

On the pad Julian scratches out a twelve-step style list of declarations.

> *Manic depression is a biological illness. I cannot make it go away because I want it to go away. But I can manage it and keep it under control. How can I do this? Take my medication and take responsibility for my treatment. No drugs or alcohol. Ever. What will happen if I follow these rules? Little by little I'll gain more and more of the independence I want and deserve.*

We negotiate what this "independence" will entail, hashing out the details, a series of punishments and rewards modeled on the five levels of privilege on the psych ward's erasable board. Except that from this point forward the "ward" will be our apartment on Bank Street. Sally's demands are desultory and unclear, as if the idea of leaving the hospital is unreal to her. The immediate future doesn't exist, only the fantasy future of perpetual childhood and genius—Sally's ultraviolet utopia. "Okay, okay, I'm sick!" she says, and with an abrupt, almost cheerful flourish she signs the contract and slides it across the table in my direction. I sign it too, as do Pat, Robin, and George.

Aaron abstains, in order to maintain his status as Sally's "peer and confidant."

We shake hands like diplomats. Sally will be discharged at 10:00 A.M. tomorrow. The Wellness Contract, with its grade school wording, is what we have to guide us.

1) *Visits at home of fifteen minutes with one friend at a time.*
2) *Trips outside of fifteen minutes in the neighborhood on my own.*
3) *Longer visits with a friend at home.*
4) *Longer trips in the neighborhood on my own.*
5) *An overnight visit with a friend at my home.*

If I am trustworthy and continue to recover, I will be able to move to the next step, one step at a time. If I am not trustworthy, I will move backward.

"Attach it to your refrigerator door," says Julian. "Try to be patient. You're doing everything right. Do you want to go home, Sally?" he asks.

Sally nods abstractedly. Then she laughs, a clipped staccato eruption, her eyes magnified and shiny, yet narrowed in their new menacing way.

We head back to Sally's room at the far end of the ward.

"I don't like Julian," says Robin. "He gives me a creepy feeling." George takes her arm. We pass a long row of half-open doors. "Now I understand why we couldn't handle Sally when she lived with us in Vermont," she says.

When we reach her room, Sally announces that she wants to be alone with Aaron.

The rest of us wait in the hall, George and I smiling helplessly at each other, Pat silent, Robin teary and warm. She's thinking of buying their neighbor's horse, she tells us. "She's a chestnut, a Morgan, just like Pepsi," she says, naming the horse that her parents kept on their Vermont property when I first met her.

"I'll have to build a stall for it," says George.

Aaron emerges from the room with Sally, his arm draped around her.

"I love my brother," she says. "My big brother. He still has a chance."

"I sure as hell hope so," says Aaron.

Sally goes back into her room. "Leave now. I want to be alone."

We say our good-byes. George will have to return to Vermont tonight, but Robin offers to remain in New York for a few days.

"I'll stay with my aunt and uncle at Westbeth, if you think it will help," she says. "It's only a few blocks away from you."

"That will be great," I say, surprised and moved.

Pat concurs, softening.

"It's not all on your shoulders, Pops," says Aaron. "You won't have to deal with this alone. You have all of us."

Robin nods with feeling, and she and George depart on a wave of good cheer.

Fabulosa, wandering along the hall, spots Aaron and, with a wild cunning, swoons dramatically to demonstrate her infatuation with him. She lifts her shirt, showing snatches of a raw and violent nakedness.

Aaron plays along, instinctively kind, even though he seems jittery and baffled.

"It's not what I imagined," he says later.

But what did he imagine? I think of the blizzard of images that I've stored about madness, the lore of lunacy that I brought to the ward when Sally was admitted, as vivid and unreal as the ogre in the forest or the wolf at the door.

"Sally is a mental patient, Pops. There are people who if they find this out will see her as an *eternal* mental patient and nothing more. They'll trust her less. I know how they talk, especially about girls. There's no mercy. They'll snicker about her and crack jokes. We have to keep this from getting out."

PART THREE

The next morning I go to the ward alone, with a suitcase into which I immediately start packing Sally's notebooks and felt-tip pens, her magazines and pajamas—the objects she accumulated during the course of her stay here.

While she changes into the blouse and jeans I brought along for her to wear outside, her roommate stirs in her bed. Her blanket slides off her like a broken layer of sod, as she sits up and plants her feet on the floor. She rises, wobbles for an instant, and then, trudging, negotiates the five steps it takes to reach the bathroom. It seems a cosmic triumph of action over torpor when she pushes open the beige steel door. And for the first time, I glimpse her face: that of a girl in her late teens, but slack and downward, as if the very muscles that sustain expression have gone dead in her.

At the nurse's station Sally's name is still on the erasable board, at Level 3: permitted to go outside for fifteen minutes at a time. Primly she sits down on the little bench near the ward's locked entrance where the classics professor had sat before his son took him home.

"You made it, girl," says Nurse Phillips. And to me, as she ducks into the glass-enclosed command post where half a dozen staff members are at work: "I'll be back in a few minutes with Sally's prescriptions."

Julian appears with information about the behavioral clinic in Washington Heights where Sally will continue to receive treatment as an outpatient after she is discharged. "Your doctor's name is Nina Lensing. I think you'll like her. I've set up an appointment for the day after tomorrow."

Blushing, he invites me to a recital in which he is to perform as cellist. "We're doing Beethoven's Opus 132, one of his great late quartets. There's every possible emotion in that piece. It's probably more than we should be taking on. But the music is supernatural."

He shakes my hand and hurries off.

I sit on the bench next to Sally and we watch a new patient being admitted, a Chinese woman in her late fifties, "hearing voices again," as the young man accompanying her calmly explains. With Rufus and another nurse, he escorts her down the hall.

Nurse Phillips returns with a fistful of prescriptions. "We don't want to see you here again, girl. You understand?"

Sally and I walk to Lexington Avenue in silence, pass through the turnstiles of the subway, and take the train downtown. Sally tries to involve the man sitting next to her in some private insight, as if he is naturally aware of what is going on in her mind. He acts interested. I move her to a seat at the other end of the car. The man—well-dressed, bearded, middle-aged—laughs, knowing and possibly nasty.

"It's dangerous to talk to strangers," I say, scolding her as if she were a five-year-old.

The apartment is empty when we arrive. On the table is a note from Pat: WELCOME HOME SALLY! SEE YOU AFTER REHEARSAL!

Sally is out of breath, having had to rest several times as we climbed the stairs, though they had never presented the slightest difficulty to her before.

A light breeze wafts in from the river three blocks away. Pat has thoroughly cleaned the apartment: everything is neatly in its place.

Sally goes straight to the shelf where the accessories of her crack-up are sitting: Shakespeare's *Sonnets*, the King James Bible, her notebooks, arranged punctiliously by Pat. Sally picks up her Walkman, handling it as one might a broken vase after a wild party.

She climbs onto the loft bed and lies down.

"Pat put on your favorite sheets for you," I say.

"Hmmm."

She slides off her shoes, which fall to the floor with consecutive thuds. When I call her name, she is too far gone to answer.

I drift through the apartment. Our harmless bohemian perch. Everything has changed, yet nothing has changed. She is ours to take care of, but she has always been ours. It hits me that I neglected to drop off her prescriptions at the pharmacy. Now it will have to wait; to leave her alone even for a few minutes is out of the question.

I telephone Jean-Paul, an independent movie producer who approached me a few days before Sally's crack-up with the idea of my cowriting a script for a young director he's promoting—a fashion photographer whose ambition is to make "a grand love story that will be an update of *Funny Face* set in the world of haute couture."

"Jean-Paul," I say to his answering machine, "I had to leave town unexpectedly. I'm back now. Let's get together as soon as possible and pick up our conversation where we left off."

I don't have much hope of this call bearing fruit, but it's a start, I have to get to work again. On the radio, Mayor Giuliani is talking to one of his constituents. "It's not the terrorists I'm worried about. Terrorists we can control. It's weirdos like you living in your caves." I turn the dial to a classical music station. A Bach sonata.

"That's like the music I listened to before you locked me up." Sally's voice drifts down from the loft bed.

With a magnetic tab I attach the Wellness Contract to the refrigerator door, like the marshal's order of seizure you sometimes see glued to the entrance of disgraced restaurants.

Manic depression is a biological illness. I cannot make it go away because I want it to go away.

I pick up one of her notebooks, with its paisley pattern on the cover—its mark of innocence—and open it to a random page:

I walk and I walk. I can't stop walking. I am by the pier. If you listen closely enough you can hear life coming from the water. The moon and stars are covered by the bright electric lights that rise into the sky—a blanket that keeps the face of heaven invisible but the world below awake. When looking up, I can see a creation of the world's future painted across the sky and the many people never resting, just working to complete that painting.

I guiltily put the book down, excusing the violation on the grounds that she is ill, her writing will tell me what I can't discover from being with her, it will help me to understand. But what have I learned, apart from further evidence of the surpassing poetry inside her?

The door buzzer rings. It's Robin. At our landing she leans on the banister, groaning comically, spent from the climb.

"Sally's asleep," I say.

But in fact she is standing behind me, having climbed down noiselessly from her bed. Her feet are bare, her face pale and shiny and, it seems to me, rounder than usual. She seems less vivid than she used to be, thickened by sleep, more stolid, yet less present, it seems, as if the live wire of her being has been grounded.

"My poor sweetheart," says Robin. She has brought taped episodes of the television show *Little House on the Prairie*. She pops one into the VCR and curls up on the sofa bed with Sally.

"You don't know how to love each other," says Sally.

By prearrangement, Robin and I ignore this, though I am encouraged by Sally's allusion to the real past, rather than an idyllic one that never existed.

"I'm going to fill the prescriptions," I say. "Then I'll be at my studio for a while. Sally's next dosage isn't till evening. You can call me there, if you need me."

It's with a feeling of hot angry shame that I hand over the full picture of Sally's mental torment to the pharmacist on Eighth Avenue: the muscle relaxant cogentin, the anticonvulsant valproic acid, the antipsychotic haloperidol, a sleeping pill, an antianxiety agent—everything she was taking at the hospital, and lithium thrown in for good measure in the event that it proves to be therapeutic.

I read judgment in the pharmacist's cocked brow as he ponders the order, though he may just be happy for the business. When he asks for my insurance information, I inform him that I'll be paying in cash.

"It'll come to $724," he says. "I'll need a deposit. They'll be ready for pickup in a couple of hours."

A flash of panic. I have $3,500 left in the bank. Pat has about $1,500.

After paying for the drugs, I walk to my little workroom, my "studio" as I call it, a boxy space in a building by the river where I have been writing, on and off, for the past ten years. Three stories of scaly white paint on a brick facade, the building stands out on West Street like a man who has quit shaving and cutting his hair. In the late 1960s, it was sliced into "affordable work space for artists," the rents kept in check thanks to the largesse of a philanthropic organization whose long-term aim was to increase real estate values in an area of tenements and abandoned auto repair and printing shops.

I haven't set foot in my workroom in twenty-four days, and the space feels different, more vacant, unnecessarily bare. The traffic two stories below on West Street echoes loudly, and motes of dust drift from cracks in the trembling walls.

From a drawer I remove the manuscript of the novel I recently completed—or so I believed. *Sleep of Reason* I called it. A disgraced big-city journalist returns to his hometown, where he lands a job as crime reporter on the local rag. He ends up writing about burglaries that he himself commits, turns his burglar into a popular figure, and then, masquerading as his creation, seduces the woman who rejected him when he was a younger man. The novel had gone to three publishers with hints of future interest but no immediate sale, and I decided to withdraw it from submission with the idea of making some changes.

Now it seems melodramatic, overromantic, my reporter self-destructive and too desperate for love.

I lay the manuscript in front of me on the desk, a crisp pile 405 pages high, neatly typed and proofed for the eyes of prospective editors. With pencil in hand, I find myself eradicating his voice—eradicating the offending "I"—and replacing it with a third-person narrator, omniscient and bloodless.

A suspicious sentence leaps up at me:

There was a hum in the air, the sonar of panic I called it, that special pitch of brutality you hear when things start breaking down.

Deleted. Along with every other passage I deem too emotional or overwrought. Any whisper of chaos that I come across in the narrative is surgically removed, each excision decided upon in an instant with no thought of its effect on the novel as a whole. It's as if my aim is to neuter the book, to relieve it of feeling itself.

I work steadily in this vein for several hours, until around five. On the river outside my window are kayakers, sail-boaters, water-skiers—a resort town scene that I gaze at as if from the wrong end of a telescope. A garbage scow floats past my window on its way to the landfill on Staten Island, ac-companied by a raucous mass of seagulls.

As I am leaving, I pass the studio of Joe, the eighty-year-old abstract expressionist painter down the hall. Joe's door is ajar, his giant box fan driving a torrid gust of air.

"How's the work going?" I ask.

"Couldn't be better!"

He hands me a mug of vodka and we listen to Joe's ancient Maria Callas LPs, surrounded by his paintings: cheerful ex-plosions of color and abruptly changing lines that are em-blematic of Joe's free spirit and hand.

At Bank Street Robin is on the sofa reading a book about the attainment of inner peace. She marks her page and hastily places it in her bag, not wanting me to see it, worried perhaps that I will disapprove. It isn't serious enough, it isn't litera-ture. I am oddly pleased; I was under the impression that she had long ago stopped caring about what I thought of her.

Sally is asleep, out of sight, the intensity of her presence as palpable as ever.

"How does she seem?" I ask.

"I think she's becoming more aware of what's going on around her. A few hours with Sally and you feel like you're speeding through a dozen changes. A dozen lives."

She slings her bag across her shoulder and starts toward the door.

"I made dinner. There's enough for you and Pat. Sally ate, then said that she couldn't breathe and would I call an ambulance. I talked her down from that. She told me that we needed to discuss our relationship, but she was going to wait until I calmed down and was myself again. It's so wild with her. I still haven't discounted the possibility that she's in touch with a higher force."

"I wish she'd get back in touch with the lower one."

"It wouldn't kill you to think positively for once in a blue moon."

As usual, our past overwhelms what the present throws up at us. We remind each other of our younger, unformed selves.

"What she needs now is love, Michael, more than ever, the feeling that she is being cared for no matter what. You know this, of course. I'm not being critical of you, it's just what I feel from her in the strongest way. I'm very sensitive to her. I have to watch myself. She gets inside me. She always has. Being with her, I sometimes feel as if I'm going to break apart myself."

I open the door. Robin lingers in the vestibule, inches from me, reluctant to leave. "She lashed out at me when I tried to give her something for her upset stomach. 'You're not my doctor!' It was hard, but I'm proud of the way I handled it. I let it slide away. I'm learning about my emotions—I wish I had done a better job of it earlier. Sometimes you have to let things float by without becoming overattached. It's a discipline. If you sit quietly you can watch your thoughts drop away like rain. If only I could teach this to Sally. It's helped me a great deal. You of all people know how emotional I get."

An hour or two after Robin has left, Sally wakes up and wanders around the apartment, half lost, trying to orient herself to her new surroundings. For an instant she rests her head on my chest. It lasts no longer than the length of time it takes to receive a peck on the cheek, and I stop myself from extracting from it the promise I am looking for. I am her father and I am her nurse, yet I've no idea what this dual role will do to us. The nurse's competence is predicated on detachment, a necessary coldness of heart.

"How would you feel if right now was the end of the world?" asks Sally.

She takes her meds without a peep of protest and tumbles into oblivion again.

I double-lock the apartment door, like Rufus.

Pat comes home churning with a muted energy, and digs into Robin's vegetable lasagna.

"I'd like you to come to rehearsal at some point," she says. "I'll let you know when we're ready. Probably in a week or two."

Sally, on the sofa, opens her eyes.

"Welcome home!" says Pat.

She rises, toppling into Pat's arms like a fallen statue.

Later, when Sally is asleep again, I say, "She's still far away. I don't see her coming back. I keep looking for signs."

"You're looking too hard, Michael."

I go back to my studio for a few hours and resume work on the sterilization of my novel.

The Outpatient Behavioral Clinic is located in an austere granite building with carved keystones over the windows in the Washington Heights section of northern Manhattan. The building is mostly devoted to treating ocular diseases, and as we enter, Sally and I nearly collide with a departing patient with a bandage as thick as a dinner roll over his left eye. In the lobby are more people in various phases of macular degeneration and blindness.

The behavioral clinic is a modest suite occupying a narrow sun-drenched corner of the sixth floor.

"Will you be okay, Father, when I'm grown up and it's time for me to leave you?" asks Sally. And she busses me on the cheek as if she has leaped into an imaginary future in which it is time to bid me good-bye.

After a couple of minutes a woman comes out to the waiting area to greet us: Dr. Nina Lensing, Sally's new psychiatrist, German-born, in her midthirties, wearing a wrinkled top with spaghetti straps, small scholarly metal-rim glasses, and a helmet of bright blond hair.

As soon as Dr. Lensing has introduced herself, Sally blurts out, "Why did this happen to me? *Why me?*"

Lensing's face opens up into a delighted smile. "I've asked the same question about myself under different circumstances a dozen times. And you know what? We're going to work on finding the answer."

Sally's leg is shaking at lightning speed.

"I bet you feel as if there's a lion inside you," says Lensing.

"How did you know?"

"Have you been pacing a lot?"

"It's all I do. When I'm not sleeping."

Lensing nimbly lowers herself into the waiting area chair next to Sally's and tells her in a tone of woman-to-woman straight talk that mania—and she refers to it as if it is a separate entity, a mutual acquaintance of theirs—mania is a glutton for attention. It craves thrills, action, it wants to keep thriving, it will do anything to live on. "Did you ever have a friend who's so exciting you want to be around her, but she leads you into disaster and in the end you wish you never met? You know the sort of person I mean: the girl who wants to go faster, who always wants more. The girl who serves herself first and screw the rest. It could be a boy too, of course, I'm just giving an example of what mania is: a greedy, charismatic person who pretends to be your friend. We may not be able to resist her every time, but one of the things we're going to try to learn is to recognize her for what she is."

"You're talking about me. I'm that girl," says Sally.

"Sally, they don't make them any smarter than you. Now come on, let's get cracking."

To me she says: "We'll spend about forty minutes alone together, then, if it feels right, I'll ask you to join us. Okay?"

"Of course."

After about half an hour, Lensing reappears, inviting me into the sanctum: a large shabby south-facing room with a ripped couch on which Sally is stretching herself and yawning, soporific yet restless.

"Your daughter is a pleasure to work with, Mr. Greenberg."

They giggle like girlfriends sharing a private joke, and I marvel at the instant rapport Lensing seems to have struck with her. Maybe she is the shaman-therapist I've been hoping for.

"Sally and I have agreed upon a goal: for her to be in shape to return to school in September. We have five, maybe six weeks. Right now, for her to try to go to school would be like running a marathon with a broken leg. So that's our first piece of good fortune: we're lucky it's summer."

Four days a week I ferry Sally to the behavioral clinic seven and a half miles up island from Bank Street. Lensing isn't always as expansive as she was during Sally's first appointment. Sometimes she's abrupt, her expression pinched, her eyes dark from lack of sleep behind her professorial glasses. A vague air of dissolution hangs over her. Her invitations to me to join them near the end of their sessions grow increasingly rare. I feel unreasonably spurned when she neglects to say hello to me or even to meet my eye. And I become almost as interested in her moods as I am in Sally's, craning my head to catch a glimpse of her as Sally steps into their room—Lensing slumped in her therapist's chair, slightly unkempt, pasty under the punitive fluorescent light, yet sharply attractive.

When she does beckon to me I feel a grateful flutter, entering with my hands held high against the sunlight which hits one in the face in that room like a thrown pie. Lensing occupies the only chair, so I am obliged to prop Sally's feet on my lap and sit down on the couch beside her. Refreshingly informal. Lensing doesn't pretend there's such a thing as a science of insanity; she doesn't lord it over me as if she harbors some secret expert power. There are no absolutes, no final authorities, she seems to be saying. We're all in the dark.

In response to my continuous anxiety about Sally's extreme medicated state, she says in her flawless, German-inflected English: "It's still a challenge for her to concentrate. No question about it. Nothing's perfect. But nothing is forever, either. Mania is . . ." Stumped for the right word, she breaks into a flurry of hand gestures as if trying to grab hold of some elusive object flying about in front of her nose. ". . . stubborn. Mania is stubborn. It hangs in there, it lays low. I'm no fan of these knockout drugs. I'll do everything I can to wean her from them. It's part of the plan."

Then she reports a setback: lithium, element number three on the periodic table and the most common mood stabilizer for manic-depressives; lithium, the plain gray salt that is the lightest solid element on earth, with its three electrons and cost of five dollars for a month's supply; lithium doesn't work for Sally.

"This is not a catastrophe," says Lensing. "It doesn't work for thirty percent of manic-depressives."

As an alternative, she is increasing Sally's dosage of valproic acid, an anticonvulsant that is sometimes effective for mania for reasons that are unknown.

"If it works as well as I hope, she won't have to swallow the bombs anymore—haloperidol, prolixin, we'll taper them off."

As a supplement, she'll supply us with tranquilizers, to be taken as needed, during bouts of insomnia and restlessness.

"I'm psychotic, psychotic, psychotic," says Sally.

"It's not an identity," says Lensing sternly.

I imagine sitting with her in a different room somewhere, without the sunshine and the torn couch and the dented radiator cover, and without Sally and the constraints of the fifty-minute hour. In the imaginary room, I am trying to charm her. Sally is forgotten. The image sharpens, and I have trouble getting rid of it, though I know I'm on shaky ground. In an effort to establish a parity of misfortune between us, I think: she's unhappy, lonely, brokenhearted. She gives more of herself than others do; she has bad luck with men. I work out in my mind that someone in her family was psychotic. It's the reason why she was drawn to psychiatry, to do battle against madness. What does she think of me, this repository of my family's woes?

I stop myself. My daughter's therapist! I tell myself I am engaged in a convoluted transference: if Lensing can heal Sally, she will be my healer too.

It is time for Robin to return to Vermont again. George and the bakery beckon. "My daily bread," she says with a yawn.

"We played Go Fish. Sort of," she says after her last afternoon with Sally. "Did you ever hear of idiot compassion? You destroy yourself by entering the suffering of others, while doing nothing useful for them."

Thin to begin with, she has lost weight, becoming gaunt,

with deep half-moon bruises under her eyes, though she claims to have napped every day with Sally, and to have slept "like a fallen tree" at night at her aunt's.

"We're at opposite ends of the energy field, you and I are, Michael. That's why we sought each other out. But we couldn't complete the promise of our polar selves, we couldn't find the wholeness we craved. Maybe Sally is the result of this failure. In the karmic sense, I mean."

With a prolonged limp embrace she bids good-bye to Sally.

August stretches before us like a desert we haven't the stomach to cross. Thirty-six days until school begins, a date that seems to belong to an unimaginable future. I worry, as Aaron warned me to, about the reaction of Sally's classmates to her altered self—the derision, the cruelty, the primal distancing that is a universal response to madness.

Sally's irate euphoria ignites without warning, in the middle of the night or at one in the afternoon. Tearing out of an unreachable stupor, she berates me for my ignorance, my fear, my helplessness, my attempt to control her, to keep her down. "I feel locked up," she says, and she doesn't only mean in the apartment—to Pat, she confesses a powerful desire to rip herself open as if she were zippered inside a fur suit.

Pat and I live in a state of red alert, monitoring her moods, her tone of voice, registering the urgency of her footsteps when she paces—at one moment her terrible indifference, at the next her ornate fantastical plans. We pass on observations to each other in a kind of shorthand, like spies. A constant wave of anxiety runs through me. If I fall asleep, I immediately wake up again, as if I am prohibited from losing consciousness for more than a few minutes at a time.

After one of her explosions, she curls up next to me on the couch, red-faced and weeping.

"I need surgery," she says.

"Where?"

"In my mouth."

The television has become the new soundtrack of our household, a frayed chorus of canned laughter, advertisements, and snowy applause, the screen flitting from one shot to the next like a traffic light that has gone out of control. Lying in front of the set, Sally seems to have decomposed. Her incapacitation enrages me. If only there was a middle ground between her explosions and this nullifying slumber. How to contain her, to activate her, to live with her now?

With election day creeping closer, Bill Clinton and Bob Dole appear more frequently on the screen, in varying degrees of damage control and ingratiation.

Dole, in California, is complaining about the Endangered Species Act: "I know all this is very important, the fairy shrimp and the kangaroo rat, but people are important too."

The audience cheers.

Abruptly I switch the television off.

Sally doesn't make a peep of protest, and I realize with a new stab of pity that though she was staring at the screen she wasn't watching it.

We follow the Wellness Contract as we would the instructions for some unassembled piece of furniture that has arrived in the mail. Julian was right—it gives us a way of measuring Sally's progress. What had seemed cartoonishly simple when we drew it up with Julian now feels intricate and complex. It would be nice to have a friend visit, even for fifteen minutes, as step one of the contract stipulates, but Sally doesn't appear to want one, and Pat and I are reluctant to allow news of her crack-up to get around.

So we have jumped directly to privilege number two: "trips outside in the neighborhood of fifteen to twenty minutes on my own." This allows Sally to sit on the stoop of our building and smoke her cigarettes, a habit she acquired in the hospital, and one that under normal circumstances we would insist she give up. In comparison with Sally's other woes, however, it seems of little importance.

During one of these cigarette breaks, a half hour passes before I notice that she has not come back upstairs. I rip through the streets trying to track her down—to the river's edge, where she spent so many hours before entering the hospital, and to the Sunshine Cafe, where the owner who threw us out that terrible day is hunched over the counter reading the sex advice column in the *Free Press*.

I finally catch sight of her at the corner of Hudson and Morton Streets, staring placidly into the window of a children's bookstore called Time of Wonder.

"Sally, were you running away?"

The question seems to perplex her. "To where?" I think I hear her ask. Clasping her hands in front of her, she peers at the images of Babar and Celeste, and the Old Lady and Zephir the monkey in their idyllic kingdom.

We ponder them together for a while, their comforting

emanations of goodness. Then I take her hand, drawing her away, past the playground on Bleecker Street, where she insists on pausing to take in the squealing delight of a group of children running through a rising arch of water pouring from a sprinkler planted in the ground.

At home, she puts on water for coffee. It takes her an eternity to raise the mug to her lips, and then it slips from her hand, crashing against the tile on the kitchen floor.

"I can't hold on to anything," she mutters. And this is true. At Dr. Lensing's suggestion, we have assigned her the chore of washing the dishes, and the shattering of dinner plates, saucers, ash trays, has become another element in the sound-track of our apartment. The dishes that survive Sally's attention we rewash when she is napping, to remove overlooked streaks of food. Her eye for details, so keen at one time, has vanished. It's as if she has been rendered half blind, groping her way through a chemically imposed carelessness.

Unable to bear waiting any longer for Sally to get out from under her pitiless ball of fire, I try to see the world as she does, and swallow a full dose of her medication.

It's around ten in the morning, and I am sitting in the living room with Sally, when it begins to hit me—in waves. I feel dizzy and far away, as if I am about to fall from a great height but my feet are nailed to the edge of the precipice, so that the rush of the fall itself is indefinitely deferred. The air feels watery and thick, until finally I am neck-deep in a swamp through which it is possible to move only with the greatest of effort, and then only a few feet at a time.

I pick up the *New York Times*, which I had bought earlier in the morning:

> Scientists studying a meteorite that fell to Earth from Mars have identified organic compounds and certain minerals that they conclude are evidence of primitive life on early Mars.

I read the sentence several times, so baffled by what the words "primitive," "meteorite," and "Mars" have to do with one another, that I start again at the first word, determined to make sense of it. By then, however, I'm lost, flailing away in my head, unable to gain any momentum of thought or meaning. The frustration reminds me of what I felt as a boy when my older brother would press his foot to my chest, holding me down. This goes on for what seems like an hour, but when I glance at the clock—and it takes another thirty seconds to read it—I see that only a couple of minutes have elapsed.

I am sitting on the couch, while Sally is at the table tapping her right foot, an expenditure of energy that seems profligate and amazing. So this is what it is to be on meds, I think dimly. Robert Lowell, describing the effects of chlorpromazine, wrote: "I could hardly swallow my breakfast because I so dreaded the weighted bending down that would be necessary for making my bed. And the rational exigencies of bed making were more upsetting than the physical . . . My head ached . . . I felt my languor lift, then descend again."

To block dopamine in a brain such as mine, which manufactures more or less normal amounts of the stuff, is different from blocking it in a manic brain such as Sally's or Lowell's. But I have the powerful sense of understanding something of what she is going through. On some fundamental level I have, like Sally, been barred from experiencing the impact of being fully alive in the world.

I rise from the couch to prove to myself that I am able to, take three steps across the room, and then, yawning uncontrollably, rush to sit down again. I make an effort to care about the simplest things—preparing lunch for Sally, returning a phone call—but an ungraspable panic comes over me, a panic of indifference, if such a thing is possible, as if I have been relegated to a bit part in the drama of my own existence and, moreover, have missed my cue to step onstage.

Gazing at Sally, I feel as if my impotence is indistinguishable from hers. I understand exactly what she meant when she said to Dr. Mason, "I feel like I'm packed in foam rubber." And I understand the allure to her of cigarettes: the stimulating flare of the struck match, the raw tingle of the smoke when it hits the lungs, the quickened heart beat when the blood vessels contract, and the narcotic lift of the nicotine. It offers its instant of actuality, of existence sharpened and in focus.

Later, when the meds have worn off and I have time to see Sally in the context of my few hours in that numbed world, I realize that the drugs release her not from her cares, but from caring itself. For caring, exorbitant caring—about the meaning of a passing glance from a stranger, the look in a news broadcaster's eye on television, the fixed fired thoughts in one's head—is the psychotic's curse. ("Skinless" is a therapist's term for those who cannot tolerate stimulation.) "To depart from reason with the firm conviction that one is following it," reads a definition of madness from an eighteenth century encyclopedia. And indeed, inordinate conviction is the chief warning sign of our delusions. For the patient to burn low, to be half asleep, to take no notice, is the medical goal—for the patient to live in a kind of emotional cordon sanitaire. Psychosis is the opposite of indifference. Indifference, therefore, would seem to be its logical cure.

Now, however, while I am still under the boot of Sally's medication, the phone rings, and I have to call upon buried reserves of energy to answer it.

I hear myself say "Hello," like someone with a pillow over his face.

"I'm sorry to wake you, but it's after eleven, *mon frère*."

"Jean-Paul," I manage to say, recognizing the voice of the movie producer with whom I left a message several days ago seeking work.

"Can we meet this morning, at my apartment?" he asks. "We have some business to talk over. I may as well warn you, I don't intend to play the usual games and hide the excitement I'm feeling. I'm almost certain you won't find it a waste of your time."

It takes me a long moment to puzzle together the meaning of Jean-Paul's words.

"My daughter is sick. I can't leave her alone," I say feebly, after an interminable telephone pause.

"Then I'll come over to your place. I'm only around the corner."

This is true. I've spent many an evening in the lavish garden of the duplex on West Eleventh Street where Jean-Paul holds court to a cacophonous guest list of fashion models, photographers, writers, and various New Age clairvoyants.

"Does it have to be today?"

"Yes. Today. Now. If you have any regard for me, Michael, you won't play hard to get." And, saving me from the arduous effort of responding to this, he announces that he will be over in fifteen minutes and ends the conversation.

In an attempt to mobilize myself, I put on the kettle for coffee, but when it whistles I am momentarily perplexed by the sound. Then I understand, though the logic required to measure and prepare a cup nearly defeats me. Before I am able to fill it with water, the cup falls out of my hand. The shattered glass looks tiny, and the prospect of getting out the dustpan and broom is as challenging to me as that of scaling a ten-foot wall. I ponder it for a few seconds, not caring. It is a picture of broken glass, not actual broken glass. It almost doesn't exist. Then, momentarily appalled at the extent of my detachment, I stab myself in the hand with a fork. It hurts! I hear myself cry out as if from across the room. To alleviate the itching rubbery dryness in my mouth, I drink straight from the kitchen tap, soaking my shirt.

The door buzzer rings, and I consider, without much concern, the picture Sally and I will present to Jean-Paul. In some muted place inside me an immense anxiety has begun to wriggle about, like a man with duct tape over his mouth, straining to be heard. I desperately need the work Jean-Paul can provide, and it is up to me to perform for it in some way, to persuade him to give it to me.

I stand on the landing and listen to him climb the stairs, a rite of passage for any visitor to my apartment, and an especially difficult ordeal for Jean-Paul, who pauses every fifteen or twenty seconds before wheezily resuming his ascent.

He appears in stages: his wiry gray hair and beard, the

spin-art splashes of burst capillaries along the corners of his sharp nose, his compact Balzacian frame huffing into view, and then Jean-Paul offering me his limp, child-sized hand to shake.

In my dullness, I allow the hand to hang in the air for an insulting amount of time, until Jean-Paul withdraws it with a frown and employs the hand to flick away the sweat that is dripping from his forehead.

"Jean-Paul," I say with the belief that I am shouting his name in welcome, yet hearing myself in a barely audible whisper.

He takes in Sally lying narcotized on the sofa, and then, after following me into the kitchen for a glass of water, the smashed cup on the tile floor.

"She's been running a fever," I explain through the epoxy of my lips. "It's been rough sledding for her—especially in this heat."

In response to Jean-Paul's expression of concern, I add, with a haste that could be interpreted as callous: "She'll be fine."

We sit down face to face at the table and I am able to pick up that Jean-Paul is uncharacteristically nervous. He has read my novel about the reporter who covers his own crimes. I completely forgot that I had given it to him, three or four months ago it must have been, in its pre-edited version, with all the unseemly emotion that I have been erasing still intact on the page.

Jean-Paul talks excitedly about the wonderful movie it will make, "a story about identity, about how we see ourselves and how we try to get others to see us, a classic movie," he says, "a *noir* but not stylized like a *noir* because that's a trap that dozens of filmmakers have lost their shirts falling into."

Trying to act attentive, I build my face into what I hope comes across as my most engaged crinkled expression, then feel the tremor of an oceanic yawn coming on, and devote all the feeble force of my concentration to keeping it from breaking the surface.

"With your permission, Michael, I would like to option the property and develop it into a film. Would you be willing, under a separate deal, to write the screenplay?"

The property. The screenplay.

"That would be . . . wonderful."

"Excellent! I'll be in touch with your agent to hash out the terms. As long as I know you're on board."

My agent. Am I still on her radar? My last communication with her was to convey my decision to take my novel off the market—a message left on her answering machine to which she never responded.

"I have to tell you, Michael, you've become so admirably calm. If I had any doubts about entrusting you with this project, they have been completely dispelled."

He rises, flushed, pleased, enjoying his sweat now, it seems, like a successful hunter or athlete.

"Get well soon, Sally," he says, and starts off on the descent to Bank Street.

After my experience on Sally's meds, I press Dr. Lensing to wean her from them even more quickly than planned. I offer the example of my brother Steve, who has ingested, by my calculation, more than six million milligrams of Thorazine over the past thirty years.

"They gave him sledgehammer doses," I say. "It went on for too long and I think it may have permanently changed him, quite apart from his emotional problems. It's true that Sally's concentration remains poor," I add, "but how can it be otherwise when the medication makes concentration impossible?"

Lensing listens politely. I become uncomfortably aware of the fervor in my voice, and suddenly feel observed, like a patient. I decide not to run the risk of telling her of my experiment with Sally's drugs. We are alone in her office and I am sitting on the couch where Sally usually sprawls, the two of us half blinded by the sunlight, Lensing with a new hairstyle, I notice, the blondness shot through with black streaks, and the tattoo of a small exotic bird on the back of her ankle which I note for the first time. Hints of her other life . . .

"I'm starting to gain momentum with Sally," she tells me after a decorous pause. "She doesn't want to be isolated, her impulse is outward, which I can tell you is extremely good news. Her desire is to be understood, and not only by us, she wants to understand herself as well. She's still attached to her mania, of course. She's remembering the intensity of her experience, and she's doing her damnedest to keep that intensity alive. She thinks that if she gives it up, she'll lose the great abilities she believes she's acquired. It's a terrible paradox really: the mind falls in love with psychosis. The evil seduction, I call it. There are things she's not telling me, I suspect, because she doesn't think I'll believe her, and she doesn't want to be disbelieved. Especially not by me."

"What sort of things?" I ask.

"Oh . . . incidents that may or may not have actually occurred. Voices perhaps."

"Voices?"

"It's a possibility, yes. Don't be shocked. It happens sometimes in cases of acute mania. The voices may be warning her not to repeat what they say. You'll think it strange to hear me say this, but I actually feel encouraged by them. They provide an opportunity for Sally to comprehend that this tempest in which she's been living was created by her."

I tell her of the plan Pat and I have made to take Sally for an outing. A day at the beach.

"That will be splendid. For all of you," says Lensing. She advises me to buy sunglasses for Sally. "You want to keep her in the shade, away from brightness. You want the sun to go down."

Laughing, she brushes something invisible from her bare arm. Starkly pale, Lensing herself appears to have gone out of her way to avoid sunlight.

"And oh, yes, be sure she wears plenty of sunscreen. Antipsychotic medication makes the skin highly vulnerable to being burned."

And so, in a rented car, we embark on our day trip, to the beach at Rockaway where I lived as a boy. Restless and volatile, Sally argues with me from the rear seat in a weaponized voice that makes my stomach turn over. "Are you monitoring my symptoms, Father? Are you inside my head?"

She leans toward me from the back of the car, her hands gripping the head rest, her mouth an inch or two from my ear.

It is more than a noise, it is *her* noise, our noise, that impostor's voice, with its pressurized bristle—how deeply I have grown to hate it!

Pat occupies the passenger seat beside me, concentrating on the book she is reading—another arcane volume to fuel her choreography, this one by the medieval alchemist Paracelsus—tuning us out.

As we are crossing the drawbridge that connects Rockaway Beach to Brooklyn, Pat says, "That's enough, Sally."

Sally fumes in silence for a few seconds, then revs up again.

I grip the wheel so tightly my hands begin to burn. I am driving slowly, plodding along, afraid to speed up, to let go. I would explode at Sally if it would shut her up, but I've learned to wait for these attacks to pass over, and not to push against them.

Pat, with an expression of infinite forbearance, returns to her book.

We make it to the beach, crammed with day-trippers like us, half-naked, dripping with salt and oil. It's the same pageant that used to thrill me in August when I was growing up in this part of town and the entire city seemed to travel to my outpost of New York, laying claim to every inch of sand—the same sand I walked on when the beaches were deserted the rest of the year.

I want to tell Pat and Sally of those summers, when, waking at just after dawn, I would set out wooden umbrellas and chairs for the paying regulars, then gather them up again at dusk, chaining them under a tarp. Afternoons, I sold Eskimo pies from a steel box with dry ice in it that I strapped across my shoulder. I was too slight for this kind of work, and I would invariably end up dragging the box through the sand, but I wanted to be out there among the show-offs and fast girls, the screaming kids in the surf, and the transistor radios blaring a competing cacophony of doo-wop, jazz, soul, and rock and roll. I want to paint a picture of that world for Pat and Sally, but it's as if I'm talking about someone who told *me* these stories, and I'm unable to capture their attention.

We trudge across the hot sticky sand until we find a space to lay out our towels thirty feet from the water. Pat continues reading. Sally takes a walk along the edge of the surf looking like Anita Ekberg in *La Dolce Vita*, with her sunglasses and high-wattage gaiety, slapping the water with her feet and flapping her arms like a bird at liftoff—an image I may once have found endearing, if overdramatic, but that I can no longer see as anything but ominous. I try to see her through the eyes of the strangers who are watching her—a girl who is unapproachable in her self-absorption, beyond sexual provocation or insult.

I collapse on the sand. Pat lies next to me, studying her book with an intensity that annoys me because I believe it's feigned. Maybe she's hoping, as I am, that order will miraculously restore itself, that what is skewed will somehow be set right. We exchange a strained glance from our respective towels. All that we used to look forward to at the end of a day—the shared anecdote, the random event analyzed and recounted, the narrative order, if not meaning, that our conversations seemed to give to our workaday lives, the jokes and arcane put-downs that were really expressions of tenderness because they bespoke the extent to which we took each other in—all the erotic, argumentative energies that supplied the frisson of our marriage have been submerged under the fallout of Sally's psychosis.

I ask her with a trace of facetiousness whether the book she is reading is interesting. "You seem so absorbed in it," I say.

"Why do I feel criticized by that observation?"

I close my eyes and listen to the hubbub of the beach, and the jetliners rumbling in and out of JFK Airport only a few miles away—familiar childhood sounds.

When we get back to Bank Street our landlord Eric is there waiting for me. A shiver of animosity passes between him and Pat as she disappears into the bedroom at the back of the apartment with Sally—to protect her from Eric's scrutiny, I'm sure.

Eric seems wrought up and peevish, and I have an idea of why when I spot him holding a copy of a literary magazine with a story of mine.

"You must be pleased about this," he says. "Why didn't you tell me?"

"I didn't give it much thought. To be honest, I'm not sure if I even like the story."

This was the wrong answer: to dismiss its importance only magnifies the imagined insult. Why haven't I done more to get *him* published is Eric's perennial complaint, though I have taken pains to explain to him that since I am not an editor I have no power to do so.

"Have you looked at my novel?" he asks.

I completely forgot about it! Yet Eric's novel is more central to our tenant–landlord relationship than the rent. He is counting on me to make a favorable pronouncement about his latest rewrite, though at a glance I could see that, like the last time he gave it to me, very little has been changed.

"I was planning to read it tonight."

He looks resentful and hurt, and I find myself thinking of my own novel which I have been slashing with the illusion that I am improving it.

"Let's go have a drink," he says.

We walk over to the White Horse Tavern on Hudson Street and sit at a table under the crude, gray, unframed portrait of Dylan Thomas, who drank himself to death here in 1953.

Eric drains his first bourbon in two gulps, and then regales me with his latest theory about his tenants: we love the address but hate our apartments, a paradox that makes us reluctant to move on even when it's a matter of personal growth for us to do so.

"My building is meant to be a way station," he says. "Eventually you have to leave. That's your moment of truth—either you have the guts to take the next step for yourself and relocate or you hang on, defeated."

I think I know what's coming, yet can't help but admire the acrobatic logic that has allowed Eric to blend his position as landlord with his higher vision of himself as the benevolent director of our lives. His tenants are the characters he really cares about, not the ones in his novel; on more than one occasion I've seen him act against his own financial interests in order to deepen his involvement with us, asserting himself as a central factor in our lives. After five years at Bank Street, my moment of truth has come: it's time for me—and Pat and Sally—to move on.

He delivers the news with the demeanor of a kind person who has been forced against his will to be harsh—grinning uneasily, avoiding eye contact, apologetic and awkward. "I'm only pointing out what you already know. It's for your own good. Anyone can see Pat's not happy here. She wants to make her own home with you, and she's right, you should. She only resents me for standing in the way."

He reminds me that when I moved in we agreed this day would come. "I'm not double-crossing you. It was part of our deal."

This is true. I'm indebted to Eric for offering me a place to live after my marriage with Robin broke up and money was scarce.

"I'll need some time," I say.

"How much time? Two months? Ninety days? Let's set a date. It's always better that way."

"All I can promise is that I'll move as soon as I can."

Eric has to defer; the timetable, at least, will be mine. Even though I have no lease, New York City's housing laws make eviction difficult. I could stir up legal hassles for Eric if I reneged on our deal, something I have no intention of doing.

We drift out onto Hudson Street and Eric immediately peels off. "I'll be staying uptown tonight," he says, mentioning the apartment of a mutual friend.

Impressive of him to have had the foresight to consider this detail.

———

Returning to the apartment, I feel a bitter tipsy pleasure at the extent to which my world has fallen apart.

"Freedom," says Sally, tapping the side of her skull. "Free-dome. Free mind. Think about it, Father."

She plugs her ears with the Walkman which she has furnished with a fresh set of batteries, and slides to the floor under the window with her chin resting on her knees.

Pat is on the phone.

I take in the partially stripped molding, the water-stained ceiling, the bandaged windows—a collage of disrepair. Our only contribution to the decor are the bookshelves I built into the walls; our other attempts to spruce up the place have been invariably discouraged. The apartment is like Eric's novel, I think, it exists as a token of the future, a perpetual possibility, incomplete and therefore unthreatened by a final verdict of its worth.

All we need to do is put our books in boxes, pack a few suitcases, and we'll be gone without a trace.

But where are we going? There is little prospect of finding a place in New York we can afford.

Pat emerges from the bathroom where she has been talking on the phone, another quirk of the apartment. It had been a bedroom previously and is large enough for a clothes dryer, a wooden bureau, and a huge bathtub with a wide, tiled ledge on which rest various books, shampoos, soaps, and candles. During its conversion, the apartment's sole phone jack was left there, next to the toilet.

"You reek of bourbon," she says. "Which can only mean that your crony isn't far behind."

"He's not staying with us tonight."

"No complaints from me on that score."

"He wants us out, Pat.

"I'm sure it was just one of your lovers' squabbles."

"It's for real. He took me to the White Horse, bought me a couple of drinks, and evicted us."

"Oh. I see."

She actually sounds pleased. In a spasm of suspiciousness it comes to me that she has engineered this in some way, nurturing her little battles with Eric, and too contemptuous of the both of us to pay her share of the "rent" in the form of propitiating him with subtly subservient gestures of friendship.

"You practically forced this to happen!"

"How? By refusing to pander to Eric like some kind of courtier? Or by expecting him to treat us with basic courtesy even if we're nothing more than squatters to him?"

"It's our home," I say miserably.

"It was never home. That's what you fail to understand." In a goading caustic voice she blurts out something about the "traumatizing" end of my "little bachelor paradise."

I slap her face, a hard nasty snap.

With a quaking, startled screech she throws a boot at my head. It hits the mark, knocking off my glasses. My head is roaring. The tensions of the summer seem to mass in me, and it is as if I am walking beside myself, hollow and enraged.

I pound the top of the table until my hand throbs, while Pat stands there watching me, smug or terrified or both, shaking her head in a *tsk-tsk* of incredulity, crossing her arms over her chest as if my loss of control proves her most uncharitable opinion of me and she is waiting for the brute hurricane either to kill her or to pass over.

The room is a blur. I grope along the floor for my glasses, then give up in a thick myopic mist.

"Look at yourself," she says.

I lunge at her, pushing her against the wall.

"Don't touch me!" she shouts, and runs into the bathroom, locking the door.

I kick and smash at it, calling for her to come out, until the panels splinter and I take each cracked piece and break it into smaller pieces and the better part of the door is lying in a pile of spearlike fragments.

Pat is sitting in the dry tub, with her hands around her legs, watching me with an odd mix of dread and anthropological detachment.

I sit down numbly on the floor for what seems like a long time. Then four policemen come panting into the apartment, in a racket of jiggling equipment, let in the door by Sally.

I've forgotten about Sally! She looks shrunken and stunned. How could I have done this to her?

Sweating in their bulletproof vests, laden with guns and ammo and flashlights and billy clubs and handcuffs and ticket books and notepads on which to write the night's crimes, the cops quickly clock the scene. Their right hands hover reflexively over the holsters of their Glock semiautomatics, while they make small talk, maintaining a casual air.

"You should tell the landlord to put an elevator in this place," one of them says to me.

"Are you going to take him to jail?" asks Sally.

"Only if he's committed a crime, young lady." And at that moment, the speaker recognizes Sally. He's the cop who removed her from the middle of the roadway on Hudson Street and brought her here with Cass. He's the one who hid the knives.

Pat is still sitting in the tub.

"Are you the lady who called?" one of the cops asks her.

She nods, and they look her over, searching for bruises, blood, marks of assault.

"She checks out fine."

I catch a glimpse of myself in the bathroom mirror, my hair wild, my eyes two bloodshot slits. I feel as if a train is running through me and sit down on the couch. Sally sits next to me, but sidles away when I try to comfort her. How can I comfort her? Her touchstone of sanity, as I thought of myself, has snapped.

"Explain your relationship to this man," one of the cops asks her.

"She's my daughter," I say quickly.

"I asked the girl. Are you this man's daughter?"

"Yeah," says Sally. "But it's not my fault."

I try to get Pat's attention, but she won't look at me. She is talking to the sole policewoman in the group, answering her questions in a voice I can't hear.

"Sometimes it's best to walk out on each other when things get too heated," says the cop who rescued Sally from Hudson Street, as he is leaving. "That's what I do. I go out and take a long walk. And if the walk lasts all night, well, that's better than doing something you'll regret for the rest of your life."

We listen to them descend the stairs, gossiping loudly, our neighbors spilling out into the hall to find out what's going on.

"Are you getting divorced?" asks Sally.

"No," says Pat.

The answer is meant for me as well. I think I detect a smile on Pat's lips, then realize that her eyes are wet with tears.

Sally slips her earphones back on and climbs up to the loft bed, while Pat and I stand in the living room like two people who have just watched their house burn down.

I'm appalled at myself, and in shock that she felt she needed armed men to protect her from me.

"Did you really think I was going to hurt you?"

"I didn't know what you were capable of or if you'd stop or even knew how. I was scared, Michael. I had to put an end to it. I didn't recognize you. It was as if you didn't care about me or even know who I was."

Her face is slightly stretched with emotion, but no streaming tears, just the telling moistness of her unnerving pale eyes.

She goes to bed, and at around 1:30 I lie down next to her.

We're like two strangers bunking together who dare not touch.

At about five, however, we wake up entwined in a stunned unconscious clutch. She quickly disengages.

"I feel sick," she says.

"What are we going to do?"

The question could refer to so many things—to where we will live, to our marriage, to Sally. Neither of us knows how to begin to answer it.

"I won't blame you if you've had it with me," I say.

"Is that an invitation for me to leave?"

"God, no."

"Maybe you think it would be easier to go it alone with Sally."

"All I meant was, this whole mess, it must seem more than you bargained for."

"I wasn't bargaining."

Her wounded imperious look reawakens a memory I have of her onstage at Bryant Park, performing a solo called *Hiding* with a buffalo skull strapped to the top of her head. Spotlit, Pat rose from under an army blanket in infinitesimal slow motion, a skeletal phoenix. The memory fills me with new feeling for her. I want to apologize, to erase last night, but under the circumstances it would seem a meaningless gesture—inadequate and too small.

Instead, I run the risk of offending her further, as I tell her that I've been sensing her misgivings, that I could feel her retreat, that I've imagined her regretting the loss of the unblemished artist's life she led before I came along, when she was content with a monastic bowl of capellini and Swiss chard at midnight. I tell her of my worry that the job of mothering Sally is more than she can reasonably accept; it will take too much out of her, she needn't darken her life with what she's not to blame for—and where will it lead, since she is not really Sally's mother and never will be, as Sally herself is so intent on reminding her?

"Do you actually think I'd bail on her? Or are you saying this because it's what you would do if our roles were reversed?"

"That's not a very charitable interpretation."

"Michael, I'm here because I want to be here. I'm worried sick about Sally."

She seems even more disappointed in me than after my outburst of last night. Apparently I have completely misunderstood her, though I could reasonably argue that she expects me to divine telepathically the withheld subtleties of her inner life, and feels let down when I fail to do so.

"I would do anything for that girl. I'm amazed that you could think otherwise."

She goes out to the living room, at a safer distance from me now.

The first light of day pushes through the window like an exhalation of white steam.

I rummage about for a large garbage bag and start filling it with the shorn scraps of the bathroom door. Part of the door is still hanging from its hinges, looking as if it has been broken open with an ax. I diligently sweep up the ancient layers of paint chips that have scattered across the floor. The pitiful after-mess of my tantrum.

"Such a pretty sight," cracks Pat.

She has made coffee for herself and is sitting at the table, not indignant or disapproving of me, as I had expected her to be, but depleted and lost. It is clear that we have passed into a new space, a flimsier, more provisional one that seems almost comically epitomized by the sheet I am struggling to hang over the bathroom doorway—to afford us a modicum of privacy until I can replace the door.

In a confessional, almost hypnotized monotone Pat is telling me about her closest friend when she was in her early twenties, a woman I have never heard of until now. "We lived together. We talked about everything. No subject was off-limits between us. She had this shining brilliance, you believed in her importance somehow, it was the most exhilarating friendship. She went mad, but it took me weeks to notice. We were too close for me to accept that anything was wrong. It wasn't unusual for us to say the same thing at the same time. And there was a point when even my dreams seemed to be a version of hers. We lived so deeply in the same world I thought her delusions were normal, they were okay—I have a high tolerance for aberrance, I suppose, we both do, Michael, or we would have realized the distress Sally was in before it was shoved in our faces.

"With my friend, it never occurred to me to step back, I was inside it with her. And when she started claiming that she had invented the alphabet, and drew diagrams on a pad to show me how she had done it—I felt destroyed. Suddenly, everything we had shared was meaningless, all our talk about art and the future and our plans—it was all nonsense."

I finish filling the garbage bag and drag it out into the hall. Then I lift out the pins and remove what is left of the door from its hinges and carry that out to the hall too.

"I want to take care of Sally and I want to get as far away from her as I can at the same time," says Pat. "When you think of how terrified and cut loose she must feel, it tears you apart. When she's her most vibrant wonderful self, she's in the most danger. That's the trick life has played on her. Just when you think you're beginning to understand her, that you're finally on the same wavelength, she says something that makes you realize you're not. You can feel how much she wants to be heard, even though it's nonsense, it's *her* nonsense, it has meaning to her. That's what I learned from my friend. I don't care if I'm not her mother. I am her mother in a way. I can give myself to Sally, like I give myself to my dance company. It's a tropism, I guess, my weakness for devotion that you like to poke fun at."

The opening of Pat's show is drawing near and her rehearsal schedule intensifies. She seems always to be rushing off to meet costume and lighting designers, or to root out props from the discount bins along Canal and Fulton Streets for the elemental Beuys-like sparseness she favors. One day five galvanized steel washtubs are sitting in the living room; on another occasion, an enormous industrial fan. She is "making movement," she says, the way one says, "I'm making money" or "making art."

She treats her dancers much the way she treats me, with a strategic elusiveness that seems to keep them guessing and off balance. She resents having to explain in words what to her seems obvious. Overhearing her on the phone, I recognize the exasperation in her voice when she tries to describe to one of her dancers the distinct characteristics of a lunge, a dive, a slide, a flop. She wants the movement to be "less nervous," she says. "But not casual." Praise is measured out in small, avidly consumed portions, like a dessert that has to be stretched to go round.

With Sally she is attentive, guiding her through her disjointed monologues, and her visions of future accomplishments and glory. "I think she's improving," Pat says to me. "But I'm holding my breath. I don't want to jinx it."

Sally doesn't mention our fight, and for a while I have the impression that she doesn't remember it, until, after I beg her to calm down during one shrill postmidnight jag, she retorts: "Oh, like you didn't almost murder Pat the other night."

Is this teasing momentary glimmer of lucidity what Pat means by Sally's "improvement"?

She paces the apartment, evil-eyed. "I'm trying to get to the bottom of who I am," she tells me.

We've grown accustomed in the middle of the night to the serrated scrape of the window when it's lifted on its rusted chain, alerting us to the fact that Sally has climbed out onto the fire escape to smoke a cigarette. I get out of bed to keep an eye on her. According to Lensing, she's not experiencing "suicidal ideation," but I can't bear to have her sit out there fifty feet above the street unwatched.

"Did you take your meds?" I ask, pestering her to ingest the very drugs I've grown to despise.

"I can't stand this! Do I seem crazy to you right now? Do I? I'm not a child. And if I was a child, I would be blessed and you wouldn't even know it!"

She dips up and down, in and out of psychosis. Neither of us knows who she will be from one minute to the next, and this lack of continuity is what is most difficult to bear. Ground down, she ceases to be an individual, not only to us, but to herself too, I suspect. There is no I, no reliable self to retreat to or upon which to stand.

The constraints my anxiety imposes on her are suffocating, but I can't stop myself from hovering over her—the jailor, the watchdog, a one-man crack-up prevention squad. I worry that in trying to calm her I am actually causing more agitation. And by the same token, when Sally tries to show me through some gesture that she is okay, I mistake it for yet another sign of disturbance.

She leafs through Shakespeare's *Sonnets*, and Yeats's poems, and the King James Bible, staring at pages she marked when she was manic, as if to recapture the feeling of the person who put them there.

"I can't read," she says. "I've forgotten how to read." And she begins to weep.

And when all should be quiet your fire burns a river of sleep, wrote Sally before the dopamine blockers erected a dam against the free flow of language in her brain.

My own mood and feelings toward her are erratic, shifting several times in the course of a day. During the worst moments, I think of her as *my* disease—the disease I must bear. In my notebook I scrawl in a furious hand: "I am intoxicated with Sally's madness in both senses of the word: inebriated and poisoned."

One morning, while Sally and I sit on the front stoop of our building, our neighbor Lou from down the street comes by walking her sheepdog. It's the first time we've seen her since her stinging retreat from Sally on the day we took her to the hospital, an incident I've replayed several times in my mind; before that day, Lou had treated Sally with a special sympathy.

My impulse is to avoid her so as to spare Sally the humiliation of being shunned again, but with a friendly overhead wave Lou comes loping across the street to greet us, pulling her mild sheepdog behind her.

"Sally! I've been thinking of you. You look so much better than the last time I saw you."

"I do?"

"You do, darling. But you must take care of yourself. Listen to your father. Now more than ever."

Sally strokes Lou's dog. "It's just like a child."

"She's *my* child," says Lou.

She obviously is aware of what happened to Sally. But how? I walk her to the corner. "Did the story get out somehow? Are people talking?"

"No one's talking, Michael. I just knew. I've lived. I know about these things."

I remind her of the way she fled from us. "Like we were lepers. It shocked me."

"All I can tell you is I know the state she was in. From my sister. My grandfather. I recognize it when I see it, and always have. I have my reasons for turning away. Now, God bless you."

When I return to the stoop, Sally says: "She's been listening to me. She can hear what I'm thinking."

By mid-August Lensing is speaking of Sally's "measurable steps toward real recovery." "Remission" is the word she often uses, to keep us from nursing unreasonable expectations.

"It wouldn't be obvious to you who are with her all the time, but it's happening. I can see it clearly."

When Sally is in the bathroom, she tells me: "I persuaded her to visit the coffee bar on Greenwich Avenue where she had some of her most disturbing moments while manic."

"I wasn't aware of this."

"She went there yesterday. During one of her fifteen-minute outings. The idea is for her to demystify these places, to see that they are ordinary, that the things she believes happened there were all in her mind. When I asked her what it was like to be there, she said, 'What kind of question is that? It's a coffee shop. I had a cup of coffee.' I loved that answer. I'm going to lower her haloperidol, starting today. If all goes well, it will be the beginning of a gradual tapering off."

"That's wonderful."

"We can't be too careful about this. The adjustment will be slow. She's still having psychotic flashes. Short in duration. Sometimes no longer than a minute."

"What kind of flashes?"

"She thinks a neighbor is watching her or that she's being followed. That sort of thing."

It occurs to me that Sally has been having these sorts of "flashes" all of her life. We just didn't know what they were. I remember Aaron teasing her when she claimed that people were talking about her on buses or at restaurants.

During the next two weeks, Lensing fiddles with Sally's medication, adjusting and readjusting her chemical regimen as if Sally is some delicate technological invention that Lensing is preparing to launch. Haloperidol is scaled back, as she promised it would be, and valproic acid is increased. At first, Sally appears even more placid than before, spending an entire Sunday in silence on the couch, forgetting even to go out to smoke.

She is now permitted to leave the apartment alone twice a day for an hour at a time. Her longer absences are a relief to both of us. We need this respite from each other.

One afternoon, she returns from the coffee bar with a

woman in her late fifties who claims to be the former Miss Georgia.

"What an absolutely amazing young lady is your daughter," she says in a homemade accent that is two parts Southern belle and one part Westminster.

Sally has already begun to emulate her speech, turning supercilious and comically patrician.

"Roseanne says I'm a midfork beauty," she says.

"That's what we call a woman who, when she walks into a restaurant, people freeze to behold her with their forks midway to their mouths," explains Roseanne. "All Sally needs to do is melt off a few pounds. She could have a splendid career as a model."

Twirling, Sally checks herself out in the mirror.

"This is not what we want Sally to be focusing on right now," says Pat frostily.

Roseanne gets the hint, delivers three loud smooches to Sally's cheeks, and hurries off.

A week, ten days pass and Sally and I are still unable to sustain a rudimentary conversation. When we do talk, it's as if we're shouting at each other across a crowded expressway: what I hear most clearly is the vast roar between us.

Then, one evening in late August, everything changes. Sally and I are standing in the kitchen. I have spent the day at home with her, working on my script for Jean-Paul.

"Would you like a cup of tea?" I ask.

"That would be nice. Yes. Thank you."

"With milk?"

"Please. And honey."

"Two spoonfuls?"

"Right. I'll put the honey in. I like watching it drip off the spoon."

Something about her tone has caught my attention: the modulation of her voice, its unpressured directness—measured, and with a warmth that I have not heard in her in months. Her eyes have softened. I caution myself not to be fooled. Yet the change in her is unmistakable.

I put on the kettle and we stand together by the stove. The opulent town house below our kitchen window is lit up for a party. Sumptuously dressed guests spill out into the yard where tuxedoed waiters carry around trays of hors d'oeuvres. A scene from *Gatsby*.

"I'm glad we weren't invited," says Sally.

The kettle boils. Sally leans toward me, resting her body against mine. "You and Pat saved my life. It must be hard for you."

It's as if a miracle has occurred. The miracle of normalcy, of ordinary existence. Following Sally's lead, I act as if nothing unusual has happened. And by all appearances, to her nothing unusual *has* happened; she seems unaware of the change.

I think to myself: I'll remember this conversation—this seemingly insignificant exchange—as the moment when Sally returned.

It feels as if we have been living all summer inside a fable. A beautiful girl is turned into a comatose stone or a demon. She is separated from her loved ones, from language, from everything that had been hers to master. Then the spell is broken and she is awake again, "surprised to have eyes."

The spell ends for me as well. My insomnia falls away and I sleep in long dreamless gluttonous sprees, unable to rise.

At Sally's suggestion we pay a weekday visit to the Museum of Natural History, and find ourselves alone among the Large African Mammals, each in its glassed dioramic world. We used to come here often when Sally was a young girl, and we relive the delight of those excursions, revisiting her favorite diorama, that of a springbok gazelle with a small bird feeding off the bugs that live in the springbok's hide.

In the museum cafeteria, she says: "I have to figure out who I am again. It's like starting from scratch."

She tells me that on the night before we took her to the hospital, with her mind blazing, she caught a glimpse of herself—"the sane me"—looking back at her from the bathroom mirror. "It was a spot in my eye, and it was there for a split second, this little part of myself that I still hadn't burned, watching me go crazy. *I see you. I know what you're doing. I know who you are.* And then it vanished." She snaps her fingers. "It didn't fade, it just went out, like the wick on one of those kerosene lamps we used to go camping with. It was like I stopped to take a last look at myself, like I was saying good-bye."

I remember the tale of the rabbi to whom a dead man came with a problem: he believed that he was alive. "Don't you know," the rabbi told him, "that you are no longer among the living? You are in the Land of Confusion." On hearing the story, the rabbi's son worried that he too was in the Land of Confusion. "Once you know that there exists such a world, you cannot be in it," explained the father.

The matter of who exactly she is now after her manic attack continues to pester Sally. At home, she asks, "Does this mean that everything I believed while I was crazy is bullshit?" How much must she repudiate? How does she sort out what she can safely keep from her mania, and what she has to discard?

Later, she wonders how something so vivid and obvious could turn out to be false. "If my insights weren't true, then what is? When you fell in love with Mom or with Pat, did you worry that it might be a delusion?"

"Only a little bit."

"But it didn't stop you."

She seems immensely matured. I realize that she has acquired another dimension. Her range of experience seems enormous. I have to remind myself of how little she has lived, that she is still a girl.

The time has come to remove the Wellness Contract from the refrigerator door. Sally goes out now for three hours alone. She is pensive, filling new notebooks, "self-educating," she tells me, "the way you did it."

We enroll her in a Japanese brush painting class at a storefront studio on Sullivan Street, so she can ease herself back into the quotidian world of conversation and simple human exchange. It proves a benign place to begin her reentry; she attends her three classes without enthusiasm, but seems heartened that they are not a total disaster.

One evening, she invites me to sit with her in the Bleecker Street playground, the site of her initial epiphany. She goes straight to a bench—"my bench," she calls it—like a worshiper to her regular pew in church. It is almost nine, no children are here, which seems to be the way Sally prefers it. "It's like visiting myself in a museum," she says.

After I have sat down next to her, she does her best to make me see it, the moment her life changed. This is where two four-year-old girls playing on the wooden footbridge near the slide signaled to her—a wave, a stare of recognition, a solemn nod—igniting the vision that had been gathering force inside her: that everyone is born a genius, but it is drummed out of us almost from the minute we open our eyes. Everyone possesses this genius. It's our unmentionable secret. When childhood is over we are afraid to salvage it from within ourselves, because it would be too risky to do so, it would rupture our drone's pact with society, it would threaten our ability to survive.

"I thought that to protect yourself from my discovery you had convinced everyone that I was insane. I really believed my vision would crush you, Dad, because you, more than anyone, were toiling to get your genius back, but you couldn't, you were trying too hard."

She takes my hand. A couple passes by, noticing us with an approving smile.

"Everything fell into place," she says. "I don't know how to describe it. My mind was going incredibly fast. But time slowed. I could see underneath the surface of things. I could see inside people. It was like I had been sleepwalking until then, waiting for this to happen."

She shakes her head in amazement and we sit in the empty playground for a while longer, in silence.

———

Dr. Lensing continues to wean Sally from haloperidol, and the change is plain to see. "She's reading again," I tell her after one of Sally's sessions at the behavioral clinic. "Her concentration is coming back."

"Let's hope it doesn't turn on her," says Lensing. "Concentration can become fixation."

But she is obviously pleased with Sally's progress. Two days later, at the end of their session, she takes me aside and whispers, "She's almost out of the woods. The dark forest."

Sally says that when she hears people climbing the stairs at Bank Street, she thinks they're coming to check on her. "Then I remind myself it isn't real. I think people are watching me, but it's only me watching myself."

Lensing warns Sally not to flirt with such thoughts. "They put you at the center of the world. They make you feel important. People are watching *you*. You feel chosen. You know better than to fall for that bill of goods."

Sally listens with her lower lip between her teeth.

"I don't know when to trust my mind anymore. I don't know when I'm being psychotic."

"When you're back at school and your life is full again, you'll be less interested in what psychosis has to offer."

At the mention of school, Sally grows tense. Only eleven days remain until she is to start tenth grade. "I won't be treated like an invalid," she shouts. "I don't want special treatment. I won't stand for it! I can do what other girls my age do!" She begins to cry.

"Where is this coming from?" asks Lensing.

To me Sally says: "Do you think I'll be able to handle school?"

I assure her that she will.

"Will my friends be able to tell that I changed?" She turns to Lensing. "If I can't handle it, I'll quit."

On Labor Day, September 2, my brother Steve calls.

"I'm not feeling good, Mikey. I want to go to the hospital. I think I've had it."

"What about those freeloaders?"

"They're gone. Junior and the others. They took off. Three days ago. I'm alone now. I swear to you. They're not coming back."

In a shaky grasping voice, he tells me that to survive he's been tramping to church basements for handout meals. "I been standing in line with the rest of the bums."

"You're not a bum, Steve. Your family is behind you. You can hold your head up. You don't ever have to be a bum."

I tell him I'll be over in half an hour.

"I love you, Mikey. Not because I have to. Not because you're my brother. You're the only one."

It has been a month since I laid eyes on Steve. After my last, disastrous visit to his apartment, with his stoned friends sprawled out on the floor, he stopped meeting me at the supermarket for our shopping dates or even answering the phone.

A week ago I received a call from a man named Edgar, who identified himself as the manager of Steve's building. "I need permission to inspect your brother's apartment," he said. "There have been complaints, and we've reason to believe Steve is violating his lease, as well as posing a health hazard to my law-abiding tenants—and to himself, I might add."

I fended Edgar off, playing for time. "I understand the problem. We're taking steps to resolve it."

"I'd prefer not to have to resort to legal action."

I reminded Edgar that he has been accepting rent from Steve since the day the building opened, twenty-one years ago. And it struck me that this was the real reason why he wanted to evict Steve: his rent is a quarter of what the apartment would fetch on the open market.

"This is the first problem you've had with my brother. Ever."

"Yes, but it's a very large problem, Mr. Greenberg."

As it happened, Edgar also contacted my eldest brother Jay at our father's scrap metal yard, which Jay and another brother, Larry, inherited after our father died.

After speaking with Edgar, Jay called me. He didn't blame him for wanting to get rid of Steve. "The way he's living in that apartment sounds revolting."

I pictured Jay with Larry in their square, gray, bunkerlike office, their metal desks only feet apart, Jay restless and hardened by a life that he fell into rather than chose.

"Tell me this," he said. "If someone was bringing drug addicts off the street into your building, where you lived, how would you feel?"

"Right now, I don't give a damn what Steve's neighbors feel."

"Well, you better start giving a damn, because they're going to evict him."

"They can't evict him."

"Bullshit they can't. The building's going co-op. He's destroying their property values."

"Steve's a legal leaseholder, with a lifelong history of mental illness. There isn't a judge in this city who would evict him, and Edgar knows it. So let's forget the threat, and figure out how to get rid of the deadbeats who are crashing with him, because if we don't, he may wind up on the street, no eviction necessary."

I told myself that Jay's callousness toward Steve was really an expression of his guilt at being lavished with Helen's love while Steve got nothing—guilt expressed as anger at the guilt-inducing party for causing so much discomfort. But what did I really know of his feelings? We were a battalion of Cains, growing up, willing to throw a weakened brother onto the garbage heap. "More for me!" was the operative ethos of our household. Cut loose by our parents, Steve became our resident scapegoat and pariah. Our shield.

"The only way to put an end to this is to scare him straight," said Jay.

To accomplish this, he and Larry planned to send a hired tough to his apartment—an ex-cop who had installed a security system in their warehouse in the South Bronx. His name was Ralph. I had met him once while visiting my brothers about a year ago, a powerful-looking, well-mannered man in tan Florsheims, a pink button-down shirt, and blow-dried hair. My brothers seemed proud of their association with Ralph. He was a testament, they believed, to the raw-knuckled world they inherited from our father (though our father never would have hired anyone to intimidate a member of his family). The idea was that Ralph would pose as a cop and threaten Steve with eviction and jail. "Wise him up."

When I protested against this tactic, my brothers reminded

me that nothing I tried thus far had worked, that fear was what people responded to, that it was for Steve's own good.

They may understand fear, I thought, but not the intractability of madness. How to explain this, however, when I just learned it myself? Steve was beyond the therapy of fear, and Ralph's threats wouldn't make a bit of difference. Steve was in another world.

When I arrive at Steve's building, Gato the Dominican doorman with a mustache so fine it looks as if it was drawn over his lip with an eye pencil, my ally in the building, is listening to the Yankees game on the radio.

"Edgar's been calling me. How bad is it?" I ask him.

Gato takes me aside. "Look, I got a loco of my own at home, it isn't easy, I know the score, you got to keep loving 'em when what you want to do is shoot 'em between the fucking eyes. Management sent orders not to let anyone up to see Steve. ¿Entiende? Some bruiser came by last week, said he was a cop. I let him go up when he showed me his badge. Otherwise, Steve's barred. Not that it changes anything. These malditos sneak in through the service entrance. They have their own keys to your brother's apartment. Tenants are freaking out, hombre. Malditos roaming around the fourth floor. People afraid to go out into the hall. People who live alone. They call me wanting to know what's up. I'm going to let you through because I know you're okay. But escúchame bien, do something to straighten out your brother, man."

Steve's door is unlocked and I walk into his apartment without knocking. Junior and the freeloaders are gone, as

Steve told me they would be, though their blankets and debris are still on the floor. They have sold his television, the cable box that Helen paid for every month, his radio, his phone. The lightbulbs are shot, and the flannel sheets covering the windows make the place feel like a cave. I pull back the sheets; a large jagged section of glass is missing from one of the windows. The room is filthy, the stench overpowering.

Steve sits on the bed, in his underwear, his cracked lower lip protuberant and slack. His skin has a calloused texture, puffy and pixilated with grime. *I know what I look like*, his expression seems to be saying. *You don't have to tell me. This is the way it is.*

"What happened to the window?" I ask

"Junior pushed this guy Raimundo against it. It was an accident. A little scuffle. They went at each other. I had nothing to do with it. Now the rain comes in. It makes me feel homeless. Can you fix it, Mikey?"

I search around for something presentable for him to wear to the hospital, but everything is dirty and torn. I settle on a striped pullover I gave him, its cuffs frayed as if they've been gnawed, and a pair of black jeans. I get him into a pair of sneakers, without laces, and we make our way to the elevator in the hall.

"I know what you're thinking. I went on the spin cycle. I went out of control. It's like Dad used to say, I can't hack it, I don't know how to have friends."

In the lobby, Steve shuffles out of the elevator like an elderly man, barely lifting his feet, his sneakers sliding off as he advances, the rear part of the shoe crushed under his bare heel.

He nods hello to Gato. "You know my brother," he says,

obviously ingratiating himself to me. "He's the one who keeps me straight. My lifeline."

Gato opens the front door for us and we step out onto Twenty-second Street. Steve immediately removes a charred corncob pipe from his pocket, jams a few twigs of tobacco into the bowl, lights it, sucks in the smoke till his face turns red, then exhales gasping. To empty the ashes, he hammers the pipe against the leg of his pants, peering at me in a burlesque of rage and contrition. "We gonna stand here all day?"

I flag a cab and direct it uptown to a hospital on Fifth Avenue—not the hospital where Sally was—I couldn't bring another member of my family there, I couldn't face them—but where our father died two summers ago.

We hurtle crosstown, the city rushing by, exhaling hotly, Madison Avenue still and pale, its window displays looking more preserved than alive, like the dioramas at the natural history museum. Another empty holiday weekend.

Steve's relief is palpable. He doesn't seem psychotic to me, but childlike and helpless. His belligerence of the past two months has drained away, spent from the effort of a rebellion that he knew from the beginning he wouldn't be able to sustain.

I ask him about the "cop" who came to see him. Steve's recollection of the visit is vague. "Was he a policeman? I guess he was. He acted like he didn't want to be there. But who would? My place isn't exactly four stars. He seemed to feel sorry for me. He told me I was going to be arrested if I didn't straighten out, I wasn't really listening, he talked like a counselor. He apologized for coming. Maybe he was shocked. I don't know. He gave me a couple of bucks for tobacco, and split."

We make it to the Emergency Room, the first checkpoint,

and settle in for a long wait on the hard plastic chairs, a television blaring overhead on its metal arm. To pass the time he recites the birthdays of most everyone in our family, including those of distant relatives, dead and alive, names I haven't heard in years. Steve knows them all with uncanny retention, though he has less to do with them than any of us brothers; on the rare occasions that he shows up at family gatherings, he slips away after an hour.

"I think you may be mentally ill too, Mikey," he says.

"What makes you say that?"

"When you were a teenager, come on, your temper, your fights with Dad." He gives me a sly, satisfied look. "They have markers for mental illness. All you need is a blood test to find out for sure. Don't take this the wrong way, I'm not trying to scare you, but I think you have it, I've seen signs. They can tell from this test if an unborn baby is schizophrenic. Because you can be schizoid in the womb too. Why do you think they legalized abortion?"

"There's no marker, Steve. No blood test. You know better than that."

He emits one of his scraping laughs.

"Come on, Mikey. I'll let you be in my dream, if I can be in yours. Bob Dylan said that."

He asks after our mother, whom he hasn't seen in many months. He's worried about her too. She's getting old. She always had Bernie. She's not used to life without him. An acid tone creeps into his voice. "She never worked, like I've worked, Mikey, putting in my time, schlepping vases of flowers in the snow." He claims that the last time he visited her, she was sitting in her apartment in the dark. Alone.

He is describing himself, of course. The person he is speaking of is nothing like our mother. Helen's apartment is unusually bright; she has dozens of friends and, since Bernie died, several suitors as well. Her phone rarely stops ringing.

Finally, a psychiatric resident interviews him. Steve doesn't protest when the resident invites me to join them. "I got no secrets from my little brother," he says.

During the interview Steve is especially wily. He obviously wants to be admitted and knows how to play his hand. He tells the resident that he is hearing voices, and I am almost certain he is lying.

"Can you identify the voices?"

"It's my sister-in-law, the wife of my brother Jay, our mother's favorite. Am I right, Mikey? Tell him. Jay got everything. He's the prince. And he got the princess and she's jabbering in my ear."

Without warning, he pulls out his tongue with his fingers and offers it to the resident for close inspection, wagging it from side to side.

"Do you see signs of rot? Sores? Cancer?"

"Put your tongue away," I say. And to the resident I explain: "He's usually shy, cleanly dressed, as gentle as the milk of God. You wouldn't recognize him."

Sparing no detail, Steve describes his exploits with Junior on St. Marks Place. I wonder if he's spreading it on too thickly as he talks about their "ho" Maxine, but he seems disoriented in a way that can't be feigned—by turns emphatic, obnoxious, innocent beyond the precincts of blame.

He is accepted into the hospital and we ride up together to the nebular safety of the locked psychiatric ward.

A nurse feeds him his medication.

"I'm a chemical experiment, Mikey. A living side effect. Remember Aldous Huxley? *Brave New World*? That's where I'm at, little brother. Soma. I started taking these drugs in 1966."

I tell him I'll be back to check on him in a day or two.

I spend the next two days cleaning Steve's apartment, throwing out the detritus of his binge, including the turntables and broken amps and computers that he and his cronies collected. I change the lock on his door, buy curtains for the windows, and hire a glazier to repair the broken pane.

During one of my trips to the compactor room I hear the metallic jingle of a chain lock sliding into its slot. During subsequent trips, I sense the eye of the person behind that door watching me through the peephole as I pass.

Finally, the neighbor steps out of her apartment and confronts me, a small soft-spoken woman in her sixties. "I know who you are," she says. "You drop some care package off for your brother and leave right away, because you can't stand to be here. But I'm here all the time, separated from him by a Sheetrock wall."

I apologize for the nuisance of the past two months and assure her that things will improve.

"You should be ashamed of yourself, letting him live like this. You obviously don't give a shit."

After three days, Steve is discharged from the hospital. He seems glad to return to his digs and pick up his life where it was before he embarked on his disastrous "social experiment," as he has now taken to calling it.

I present him with a new key, a fresh tin of tobacco, and his weekly groceries, which I have stored neatly in the fridge.

In a matter of minutes he has reinstalled himself in his Barcalounger with his pickle jar filled to the brim with Lipton's tea.

"I'm going back to work for the Greeks," he tells me. "The busy season is about to kick in. Ten, twelve deliveries a day. You'll see. High times are around the corner. I heard it on the radio. Clinton's going to be reelected president. A new boom."

On September 9 school is to begin, and as the date approaches Sally is filled with dread at the prospect of reentering the world, let alone facing her classmates. She is ashamed of what she might have done in the late spring when she was gearing up for her manic gallop. Imagining the worst, she has taken to crossing the street to avoid facing neighbors and shopkeepers whom she barely knows, convinced that she disgraced herself with them. The fact that she can't remember how only serves to sharpen her retroactive shame.

"I don't know who I was," she says. "What if people ask me to explain the weird things I did?"

"What kind of things?" asks Pat.

"I don't know!"

Robert Lowell felt that talking about a manic attack after "the froth of delirium has blown away" is like "a cat trying to explain climbing down a ladder." Sally is that cat, laboring downward after her fleet heedless climb. The vividness of mania has left her unsure of where her thoughts ended and her deeds began. It doesn't seem possible to her that the high drama of her projections weren't actual events, and that gray ordinary life went on as usual while she was mad.

"It was all happening inside you," I tell her. "No one could see it, until you boiled over with Cass. And that was already in July."

But the blank spots in her memory continue to haunt her. "I was out of my mind. But I don't know what that really means."

Lensing tells me that her anxieties are to be expected. "'Better old demons than new gods,'" she says, quoting the Chinese proverb. "The mind flies back to the storm it's familiar with. There's a certain brittleness to Sally right now. A tendency to self-manufacture stress."

She increases Sally's antipsychotic medication, though it remains well below what it was when she left the hospital. "Just for a few days, to help her over the hump," Lensing explains.

But then Sally frets that her friends will know she's sedated.

"What if I don't pass the lunch counter test," she says, referring to the ability to be in public without one's mental illness being detected.

Under Lensing's guidance she is keeping a "mood journal," chronicling, with worrying meticulousness, every shift of her heart. I wonder if she is overdoing it; shouldn't she be encouraged to look away from herself, to look outward?

Four days before school is to begin she says, "I think we're rushing it. I'm not ready. I haven't had a chance to deal with what happened. I'm sorry. Will I ever stop disappointing you, Dad?"

She plugs along bravely, however, delivering her mood reports to Lensing, though she herself harbors doubts about their reliability. She is the sole source of information about herself, and that's the rub. "I have a knack for fooling people into believing I'm in control. They go along with me, when I'm a total mess. It's a little scary."

Lensing isn't worried about being fooled. "The spectrum is narrowing," she tells Pat and me. "Her mood swings are less radical. She's an exceptional writer. It just pours out of her. She draws you in. It has . . ."—she pauses, searching for the word—". . . *immediacy.*"

She places Sally on a strict regimen, "the manic-depressive diet," she calls it, designed to keep Sally firmly planted on the ground. "As little refined flour as possible, but potatoes are okay. Lots of vegetables and protein. Two tablespoons of flaxseed oil per day, nine hours of sleep without interruption, and no naps."

Alone at dinner with me, Sally has the jitters of a bride just before her wedding, unsure of whether she is throwing in her lot with the right man. "I can't go through with it. Why don't we just accept the fact that school is something I can't handle."

"Have you considered the possibility that things might work out?"

"Possibilities don't help me. I need to know."

"No one can be sure about the future."

"Yes. But it's different with me. If my mind turns on me, I won't even know it's happening. I won't know I'm being a freak. But everyone else will."

I think: how fragile she is. Yet the unstoppable force of her being is the opposite of fragile. I wish I could stop her from overidentifying with her illness, but how can I when the very mechanism of managing it requires a self-scrutiny that constantly reinforces it in her mind?

When I suggest that she take it slow and wait a few more weeks before starting school, she says with horror, "And be a dropout? Are you serious?"

Around midnight Pat returns from rehearsal. Sally has gone to bed. Pat sits down a few feet from me on the couch, silent and intense. It's been almost a month since our blowup, and we are still tentative with each other, halting, careful about what we say, and physically shy. It's as if we've been waiting for a new order to declare itself, a new way of being that we know instinctively not to force along.

Pat sits with her knees pressed together, on the edge of the couch, as if she's about to spring up at any second. I put down the book I've been reading.

"I think we should have a child," she says.

It is clear to me that this is not a suggestion, that Pat has already made up her mind, and my first overriding impulse is to argue against it. Would it be wise for us to do such a thing now? Shouldn't we wait at least until we're resettled? Eric is impatient for us to move, nudging us out the door with a steady stream of hints and unpleasantries. And although we have spent the better part of each weekend looking for an apartment, we've yet to find one we can afford.

"Can we handle a baby when everything is so uncertain?" I ask.

"Things are always uncertain," says Pat, inadvertently paraphrasing the platitude I delivered to Sally earlier in the evening. She brusquely rises, obviously offended.

Overhearing us, Sally climbs down from the loft bed,

stricken. "I knew this would happen. You'll never love me as much as your own baby. It's the biological law. You'll say you do, but it will be a lie, not because you want to lie, I don't think you ever lie, Pat, but you won't be able to help yourself, I'll always be second."

She sits on the couch where Pat had been sitting, her feet curled under her, wide awake, worrying.

"Pat will be an amazing mother," she says to me in a whisper, so as not to be overheard.

During the weekend we visit friends in Woodstock in upstate New York. They have a healthy five-month-old baby girl. Sally grasps her fists and talks quietly to her, and our friends remark at how absorbed and tranquil the baby is in her presence.

At lunch, the new father props the baby in his lap and his wife trains a video camera on the scene.

Impulsively, I jump up from the table, throw my arms around Sally, and say, "This is *my* baby. Video us too!"

Sally turns her head away, and Pat gives me a scalding look from across the table.

"One is always a baby to one's parents," says our hostess kindly.

She turns the camera on us for a few seconds before politely putting it away.

I sit down, burning with shame.

The night before school is to begin, Sally is supernaturally calm. She is annoyed at the fuss Pat and I make as we prepare her for the big day: a special compartment in her backpack for her noontime meds, and a note to remind her to take them.

In the morning, Sally makes fun of my checklist of "things to remember."

When I ask her if I'm being overprotective, however, her sarcasm dissolves. "God, no. I'm terrified. That's the problem. I need this."

The familiar simmering apprehension comes over her. "What am I going to say when people ask what I did over the summer?" She throws her voice into a high-pitched mimicry of chitchat. "'Oh, I spent July in the loony bin. I found out I was psychotic. What about you?'"

I advise her to keep the events of the summer to herself. "People won't understand. Or very few will. You don't know what kind of prejudice you'll run into. Best to work it out with us, and with Lensing."

But am I right about this? Is it really better for Sally to conceal what happened? It may not be possible. And what of the burden such a secret will place on her?

Too preoccupied to work, at three o'clock I'm sitting outside on the stoop waiting for her to come home.

"How did it go?"

"Fine," she almost snaps. Then, in a softer voice, "I didn't get eaten. No one ran away from me or noticed anything strange, except that I gained weight. But everyone looks different than last year."

We celebrate at dinner. Robin phones to congratulate her. Then Aaron calls to cheer her on. "Nothing happened!" he says triumphantly. "Never have those two words sounded so good."

To be congratulated for nothing is "pathetic," insists Sally. But I can see that she is pleased.

The school week ends and nothing continues to happen.

Lensing pulls back the antipsychotic medication again, and by the end of September Sally is only taking a tiny dose before bed. Her lightning wit returns—her verbal precociousness, and her intense feeling for people, including those she encounters in literature and in movies.

She forms a tight group with three girls from her class, and often, after school, they happily colonize the apartment. Evenings, I listen to her on the phone with them, intimate, biting, gossipy—the buoyant sound of health.

After a long discussion with Pat and me, she tells them about her crack-up. They readily accept the news. Being an alumna of the psych ward confers social status on Sally. It's a kind of credential. She has been where they have not been. It becomes their secret.

On October 23, the day before the opening of her dance performance, Pat calls me late in the afternoon. "Tech rehearsal was a disaster," she says as if what she suspected all along has finally been confirmed. "The piece looked terrible. The dancers forgot everything I taught them. They started posing, moving in time with the music. It was deadly." She apologizes for not inviting me to rehearsal as she had promised. "I realized you were too close to the material. You wouldn't be able to see it with your best critical eye."

She hasn't told me anything specific about the piece, and I have the sense that she dreads showing it, though this may be just her normal pre-opening night panic.

At home, she confers with the dancers for hours by phone.

"They need to be a little scared," she tells me. "There's no compromising now."

The living room floor is covered with sheets of tracing paper—Pat's latest prop. I hear her cutting the paper as I drift off to sleep.

At 5 A.M. she is sitting on the edge of our bed, pale with apprehension.

Good news: the show is sold out. I arrive with Sally and watch the audience drift in with a sharp expectant rush. The seats around us fill. The chatter grows louder. I spot Helen wearing a purplish dress woven to a brocaded finish. She embraces Sally, introducing her to the two friends she has brought along as "my gorgeous granddaughter."

"Congratulations to the husband," says one of Helen's friends. "You must be very proud."

Sally grips my hand. I feel a triple panic: hers, Pat's, and mine.

"Pat is so brilliant," Sally says, after my mother and her friends have gone off to their seats. "She held on to her creativity. I feel so lucky that she loves me. I do believe she does. Do you think she does?"

The house lights go down and we are plunged into Pat's psyche, but also, astonishingly, into a mirror of our own. *Clinical Data* the piece is called. The dancers lunge and flop, jerky and raw, while two actresses follow them spouting poisoned rapid-fire phrases—". . . we're here to take out the useless parts of your brain . . ."—their haunted whispery voices overlapping. They're the voices inside the dancers' minds.

Sally seems mesmerized. I watch her watching: her still face and large black eyes. The dancers look as if they have been caught by surprise, ungainly and vulnerable within their invented world. The tracing paper that Pat had been cutting in our living room the night before has been assembled into fifteen dresses which hang on fishing lines from the rafters, each with a yellow sash. An enormous fan, its steel blades glinting, sits upstage center like a bull's-eye.

The fan is switched on, blowing almost violently through the theater. The dresses have a feathery look suspended in midair. The dancers slip into them, the paper rustling loudly as they move, crumpling on their bodies and falling off in shreds that sail randomly around the stage. The effect is of sloughed skin, as the dancers in their torn dresses assume a ravaged, fashion catwalk appearance. The action may be taking place in a prison from which the effort to escape is comical, because even when they think they have broken free the dancers are still there.

"What's your diagnosis?" asks one of the voices, the way a prisoner might ask, *What are you in for?*

A Colombian saxophonist, whom Pat met while he was playing for quarters in the subway, plays boleros he composed. The dancers blow bubbles at each other that land like psychic bombs. It comes to me that we are in the dayroom of the psych ward, reimagined as a kind of lunatic ball.

So this is what she has been doing all summer, I think. I have the urge to get up and leave. It's too intense. I take Sally's hand. She seems delighted and amazed.

When it's over, the audience is momentarily stunned. A few seconds pass before the applause gathers momentum.

The dancers take their bows, spent and euphoric. I glance at Pat, standing in the back of the theater, her face swollen from lack of sleep, cheering for them with her hands over her head.

Helen congratulates her on her way out of the theater. "You captured it, Pat. You showed us something profound." She embraces Sally again. "There was a lot to think about out there tonight, sweetheart. But don't think too hard."

Her friends seem bewildered and moved. "She's a quiet girl," I hear one saying of Pat as they head toward the exit. "A lovely girl. You don't expect this from her."

At home, Sally says, "It was like watching my episode from the outside. It was beautiful. You showed it to me. I just hope we didn't scare anyone. All those people in the audience, I mean. And how they were cheering for you, Pat!"

She attends the second performance, hanging around the dancers afterward, sitting backstage next to Pat with her head in her lap.

Two weeks later, she receives an A—her first ever—on a paper about James Baldwin's essay *The Fire Next Time*. "He wrote this book so he wouldn't go mad," she tells me.

The shelf on her loft bed is piled with new books she has acquired: *Women and Madness*, *The Myth of Mental Illness*, *Is There No Place on Earth for Me?*

Sometimes, after school, she retreats to her loft bed or takes long wandering walks in the Village. I can sense her contending with what she knows is inside her now, bewildered and brave, negotiating with it, as if trying to reach a truce with herself.

In December the three of us move into an apartment of our own on West 108th Street, and the time of our troubles limps to an end. At least for now.

POSTSCRIPT

Two years later, in December 1998, Sally was in the birthing room with Pat and me after her half-brother Brendan was born. She worriedly comforted Brendan when he whimpered under the warming lamp in his bassinette. She adored him when he was little, whispering in his presence when saying something she believed he was too tender to hear.

In June 1999, Sally graduated with honors from high school, and in September she started classes at a small liberal arts college in Manhattan while continuing to live at home. She seemed to have entered a period of intense creativity, catching her teachers' attention with her writing and her original turn of mind. But in the spring she had to withdraw from school, beset with manic psychosis after being free of it for more than three years. A series of hospitalizations followed. It took nearly a year for her to find her footing again.

In 2001 Sally became romantically involved with a former high school classmate, Alex. They were each other's "first," as Sally put it. "He told me he loved me," she said, over the moon with him. It seemed a huge leap forward. They were relaxed with each other, Alex eager and innocent, the two of them quick to laugh, sharing private jokes and myriad points of connection. They seemed considerate and protective of each other, and though Alex was aware of the medication Sally was taking and what it was for, he seemed as mystified by the deeper currents of her illness as I once had been.

Sally moved in with Alex during his last year of college in upstate New York, working with young children at a local day care center, and at the college dining hall in order to help Alex make it through to graduation.

In July 2004, they were married on the shore of Lake Seneca in Geneva, New York, with families and friends in attendance, and Brendan carefully bearing their rings on a small white cushion.

Two years later, for health reasons, Sally was taken off Zyprexa, the powerful neuroleptic that had replaced valproic acid as her main medication, and that, despite several undesirable side effects, had helped keep her out of the hospital for more than five years. Psychosis jumped to life in her with renewed force, as if it had been lying in wait.

In the summer of 2007, she separated from Alex. She now lives in Vermont near Robin and George. She works part-time at Robin's bakery, specializing in the confection of lemon squares and muffins. She also helps out at a nearby farm, tapping maple trees for syrup and tending to the goats and cows. We talk almost every day, Sally wry about herself, and courageous even during her periods of retreat and loss. She is determined to learn to anticipate her worst bouts of psychosis, and head them off before they overwhelm her. "I'm trying to recognize when it's coming on," she says, "so I can get out of the way or at least drop to the ground like you would when caught in the crossfire of a shootout."

When I told her I was writing a book about the summer of her first crack-up, she said, "I like the idea that you're thinking so much about me." Then, after pondering it for a while, she added, "I want you to use my real name."

AFTERWORD

Ten years have passed since the publication of *Hurry Down Sunshine*, and the question that readers invariably ask me is, "How is Sally doing now?" My truthful answer is that she lives an engaged and purposeful life, brimming with rich relationships. In the best of times.

But manic depression is a lifelong affliction, and Sally has no choice but to contend with its unpredictable, sometimes gale-force winds. She has become vigilant of the galloping thoughts that are often the precursor to psychosis—the beguiling insights, the imaginary voices that drown out real ones as they beckon her toward the thrill of their alien world. Aware of the danger, she will increase her medication and retreat into long bouts of sleep, the better to combat the gathering force inside her.

Occasionally, the wind is too strong to resist and sweeps her away. A stint in the hospital will follow, and then the hard work of reassembling her psyche so she can return to the world she temporarily left behind. To me, this is Sally's most heroic undertaking. The temptation to give up, to cry "Why bother!" and tumble into a listless, post-psychotic depression is enormous. For a short time Sally may succumb to this temptation, but before long she will commence the process of rebuilding herself, like someone shoring up a repeatedly battered wall.

She does this so as not to lose or destroy the relationships she most cares about. Sally's talent for friendship, her empathy and open, generous nature have protected her as much as any medication.

In December 2015, she married a young man in a small Episcopal church next door to Robin's bakery in Vermont. The wedding was modest, their vows exchanged with certainty, their voices barely louder than a whisper. Time and again, I have been awed by their calm devotion to each other, their steady, unobtrusive love.

An astute observer, Sally's husband has acquired a deep understanding of her illness. Together, they neither minimize nor exaggerate the role it plays in their lives. Manic depression is a presence in their marriage, but it is only one presence among many others.

They live now in Massachusetts, where Sally's husband teaches high school biology and Sally studies early childhood development with the hope of working one day with young children.

They want a family, but with Sally's regimen of medications and the possibility of a serious postpartum depression, they have decided that the risks of pregnancy are too high. They are in the midst of planning to adopt a child.

September 2018

ACKNOWLEDGMENTS

I am indebted to Judith Gurewich, publisher of Other Press, whose editing skills and unwavering commitment to this book nourished it throughout; and to Jim Campbell for his keen reader's eye.

Quotes from Robert Lowell come from Ian Hamilton's *Robert Lowell: A Biography* (New York: Random House, 1982). It is both a superb account of the poet's life and a harrowing depiction of mania during the course of a lifetime and its effect on those who find themselves standing in its path.

Richard Ellmann's classic biography *James Joyce* (New York: Oxford University Press, 1959) and Brenda Maddox's excellent *Nora: The Real Life of Molly Bloom* (New York: Houghton Mifflin, 1988) provided the essential outline of James and Nora Joyce's troubled relationship with their daughter Lucia.

Michael Greenberg's memoir, *Hurry Down Sunshine*, has been translated into eighteen languages and was named a best book of the year by *TIME*, *Library Journal*, and Amazon.com. A collection of his essays, *Beg, Borrow, Steal: A Writer's Life*, was published in 2009. From 2003 to 2009, Greenberg wrote the "Freelance" column in the *Times Literary Supplement*. From 2010 to 2012 he was the author and creator of "The Accidentalist" column in *Bookforum*. He teaches writing in the MFA program at Columbia University and is a frequent contributor to the *New York Review of Books*.